YOUR
BODY
KNOWS
BEST

Other Books by Ann Louise Gittleman, M.S.
and Certified Nutrition Specialist

BEYOND PRITIKIN
BEYOND PRITIKIN, REVISED AND UPDATED
SUPER NUTRITION FOR WOMEN
GUESS WHAT CAME TO DINNER: PARASITES AND YOUR HEALTH
SUPER NUTRITION FOR MENOPAUSE
SUPER NUTRITION FOR MEN

YOUR · BODY · KNOWS · BEST

THE REVOLUTIONARY
EATING PLAN
THAT HELPS YOU ACHIEVE
YOUR OPTIMAL WEIGHT
AND ENERGY LEVEL FOR LIFE

Ann Louise Gittleman, M.S.
with James Templeton and Candelora Versace

POCKET BOOKS

New York   London   Toronto   Sydney   Tokyo   Singapore

The author of this book is not a physician, and the ideas, procedures, and suggestions in this book are not intended as a substitute for the medical advice of a trained health professional. All matters regarding your health require medical supervision. Consult your physician before adopting the suggestions in this book, as well as about any condition that may require diagnosis or medical attention. In addition, the statements made by the author regarding certain products and services represent the views of the author alone, and do not constitute a recommendation or endorsement of any product or service by the publisher. The author and publisher disclaim any liability arising directly or indirectly from the use of the book, or of any products mentioned herein.

POCKET BOOKS, a division of Simon & Schuster Inc.
1230 Avenue of the Americas, New York, NY 10020

Gittleman, Ann Louise.
  Your body knows best : the Revolutionary Eating Plan that helps you achieve your optimal weight and energy level for life / by Ann Louise Gittleman with James Templeton and Candelora Versace.
      p.   cm.
  Includes bibliographical references.
  ISBN 0-671-87592-2 (hbk.)
  1. Nutrition. 2. Nutrition—Genetic aspects.   3. Nutrition—
Requirements. I. Templeton, James William. II. Versace,
Candelora. III. Title.
  RA784 G54   1996
  613.2—dc20   95-33222
                                                         CIP

First Pocket Books hardcover printing March 1996

10 9 8 7 6 5 4 3 2 1

Text design by Stanley S. Drate/Folio Graphics Co. Inc.

POCKET and colophon are registered trademarks of
Simon & Schuster Inc.

Printed in the U.S.A.

For those who do not follow where the path may lead but go instead where there is no path and leave a trail

Acknowledgments

A book materializes because of the support and encouragement of many devoted individuals. I would like to gratefully acknowledge the following associates and friends who have been there for me and my message:

Thank you to my first editor, Denise Silvestro, and to Amelia Sheldon, my second editor at Pocket Books, for their excitement and belief in this project. Kudos to Melissa Diane Smith, who assisted me so graciously in making last-minute additions and updates to the manuscript. And as always my appreciation to my literary agent and dear friend, Michael Cohn.

Very personal thanks to the following professionals who have inspired me and helped me through their own unique work: Bill Wolcott; Pat Connolly; Dallas Clouatre, Ph.D.; Nicholas Gonzales, M.D.; Julian Whitaker, M.D.; Jane Heimlich; Linda Lancaster; Hal Huggins, D.D.S.; Hazel Parcells, Ph.D., N.D. and D.C.; Nathan Pritikin; Carlton Fredricks, Ph.D.; Ronald Hoffman, M.D.; Weston Price, D.D.S.; William Donald Kelley, D.D.S.; Melvin Page, D.D.S.; Robert Crayhon, M.S.; Deepak Chopra, M.D.; Lendon Smith, M.D.; Dick Lamb; Bruce Barlean; Roy Speiser, D.C.; Alexander Schauss, Ph.D.; Mark Anderson; Allen Kratz, Pharm. D.; Patti Hausman, M.S.; Donna Wild; Royal Lee, D.D.S.; Terry Lemerond; Julia Bondi; Kathryn Arnold; Peg Jordan; Karolyn Gazella, Siri Khalsa, and Linda Clark.

Contents

Introduction

As a nutritionist, I'm concerned. No, make that worried. Really worried. So many women are doing everything they're supposed to do—exercising like mad, cutting the fat, and increasing those high-energy carbos in their diets. Women are being told they can eat whatever they want whenever they want it, as long as the food is high in fiber and low in fat. What worries me is that many women are not losing weight at all on this regimen, and even worse, they're complaining of increased weight gain, tiredness, and uncontrollable sugar binges.

The truth is, not everybody can handle a diet so low in fat and high in carbohydrates. Women especially can have trouble on such a diet. I found when I myself ate a high-carbohydrate diet, I was constantly hungry and never satisfied. I ate Grape-Nuts for breakfast, a sandwich of vegetables in pita bread for lunch, and a pasta dish for dinner. I ate no red meat, a little chicken, and no salad dressings or butter. I was constantly looking for nibbles between meals, and often tried to fill up on frozen yogurt, wheat crackers, rice cakes, and other carbohydrate-based foods. In fact, the more carbohydrates I consumed, the more I craved. If you have found this to be true for yourself, rest assured, you're not alone.

You've probably tried more than one version of the low-fat, high-carbohydrate diet yourself. You've fretted over fat grams.

You've perused Ornish and were no doubt relieved when you heard you could eat more and weigh less. You've even been motivated by former fatties who want you to stop the insanity of dieting. Most likely, you not only didn't lose weight but you saw your best friend on the same diet lose 15 pounds with ease. Why is it that one diet can work well for one person but not another? It's not because you didn't follow the diet correctly. It's because the diet didn't follow you! What do I mean by this? Simply put, each of us is different in so many ways, there is no one diet that is suitable for everyone.

From Fit for Life to Scarsdale; from macrobiotics to Slim-Fast; from Atkins to Pritikin—there seems to be no end to the well-intentioned advice of diet gurus who believe their own single specific dietary plan will be the answer to *everyone's* problems. Even with all this advice, millions of Americans are still battling weight problems as well as high cholesterol levels and the threat of heart disease. Many of us have relied so heavily on the currently popular low-fat, high complex-carbohydrate, low animal-protein diet as a guideline that we've also developed a host of low-grade symptoms that keep us from feeling healthy, strong, and vital.

Each of Us is Unique

By focusing so strongly on the idea that one diet will provide all the necessary nutrients for everybody, we've completely ignored a primary factor that governs all living beings. Each one of us is different, from the shapes of our bodies to the color of our eyes, from the color of our skin to the texture of our hair, from the part of the world that our ancestors have come from to the ease or difficulty with which we gain and lose weight. We have different tolerance levels for different foods: fully 70 percent of the world's population suffers from the inability to digest lactose (milk sugar). We have various physical limitations and inherited tendencies that can result in diabetes, high blood pressure, and heart disease, all of which can be aggravated by the wrong diet. All our differences play a part in our "biochemical individuality," a term coined in the 1970s by the late Dr. Roger J. Williams, a biochemist at the University of Texas at Austin.

We have different kinds of jobs and life-styles, various tastes and preferences, strong likes and dislikes. Age and activity levels impact each of us differently, and even gender has a strong influence on our metabolism. Although we all may be created equal, the truth is that biologically, men and women are different. Men can lose body fat much more quickly than women, even when they both engage in the same amount of vigorous exercise and watch their diet. That's because the more muscle we have, the easier it is to burn fat. The male body is made of more muscle and lean body tissue, thanks to the male hormone testosterone, whereas the female body, due to female hormones such as estrogen, has a greater buildup of body fat.

In attempting to create a one-size-fits-all diet plan for all of us, we've lost the sense of our own uniqueness. The fact that we've failed to take into account that different people have different dietary needs has played needless havoc on our health as a population and as individuals. In addition, many of us have lost the simple joys to be found in eating, the sensuous pleasures of taste, texture, and aroma, and the social aspect of making and breaking bread with family and friends. They've been replaced by the mental stress of keeping track of fat grams and calories, not to mention the emotional stress of guilt when we stray from our self-imposed dietary rules and restrictions. We've even forgotten some of the common sense wisdom our mothers taught us. It seems almost painfully old-fashioned to think of a healthy diet in terms of eating three balanced meals a day, in which all components are eaten in moderation (and not too heavy on the starch, remember?).

What all of us are missing in this glut of information may be the very key to our dietary woes. The answers are almost deceptively simple, but they have come to me after 20 years of extensive research, experimentation, and personal and professional experience. The truth is, *there is no one diet that works for everyone.*

Three Important Factors to Consider

There are several factors that I will be talking about in this book to help you determine the perfect diet for you: your ancestry and genetic heritage, your blood type, and most importantly, whether you are a **fast burner** or a **slow burner.** If you have a revved up motor and burn food off quickly, you should be eating different foods than a person who is slow and steady. The *slow burner* has her own specific dietary recommendations that will help her speed up her metabolism and, in so doing, burn off accumulated fat.

Blood type and heredity also play important roles in how to determine the ideal diet to promote your best health. I first began to suspect that blood type should play a greater role in a person's diet when I was doing research for my book, *Guess What Came to Dinner: Parasites and Your Health.* During my fact-finding mission for the book, I was fascinated to read again and again that blood type A was a risk factor for infections caused by *Giardia lamblia,* one of the most common waterborne parasites today. Many individuals who have this blood type have a genetic lack of hydrochloric acid digestive enzymes that makes them more susceptible to developing the ailment. Because our blood type is an inherited factor that influences some aspects of our health (like giving us more of a tendency to develop parasite infections and other conditions), I went on to explore how blood type could be a determining factor in selecting the correct diet for each of us.

This compelled me to begin searching for other elements that would further personalize diet. My search led me to the over-looked but well-documented fact that maintaining a diet as close as possible to the diet our ancestors ate is crucial for maintaining our optimum health. Ancestry, then, in addition to metabolism and blood type, became determining factors in helping me develop the best diet for myself and for my clients. Now you can use this same information to design the most favorable diet for you. Being aware of these three factors and how they relate to you personally will help you choose exactly the right kind of foods—or fuel mix—to eat that will help you lose weight and gain optimal health and well-being.

Much of what you will be reading about food in the following chapters is different from—and in some cases contrary to—what you've been hearing for the past several years: fat is bad, carbohydrates are good, and all red meat should be avoided. Nutrition, as you will learn, is not so black and white. The truth is that much of the information in this book, which will be new to many of you, has been around for a long time. The term *biochemical individuality* is at least 20 years old, and the concept of individualizing dietary needs can be traced back to antiquity. This information has been lost or ignored by fat-phobic nutritionists who focus diet plans on one aspect of proper food intake.

My Quest for the Right Diet

Sorting out the truth among all the conflicting dietary information and presenting it to the public has been my life's work. In addition to all my studies and my professional positions, I have been busy using myself as a guinea pig, trying out every new bit of dietary wisdom on myself. I've been through the same ups and downs many of you have, including bouts with weight gain while on the diets that promised otherwise.

From my early studies at the New York Institute of Dietetics and the master's degree program in nutrition at Teacher's College at Columbia University, through the years I was Director of Nutrition at the Pritikin Longevity Center in the early 1980s and the past decade of my own research with thousands of clients, I have consistently studied whatever current information I could find relating to health and nutrition.

In addition to my academic work, I expanded my realm of experience to include working with other health care professionals, which has been an important adjunct to my ongoing education. My experience as chief dietitian of the pediatric clinic at Bellevue Hospital in New York and as a bilingual staff nutritionist for the USDA's Women, Infants, and Children food program at Hill Health Center in New Haven, Connecticut, gave me an appetite for researching medical reports that continues to be a strong part of my work today.

My background and training have been conventional, clinical, and academic, but I always remain open to nontraditional alternatives that prove workable. As author of *Beyond Pritikin* (Bantam, 1988), *Super Nutrition for Women* (Bantam, 1991), *Guess What Came to Dinner* (Avery, 1993), and *Super Nutrition for Menopause* (Pocket Books, 1993), I have explored in depth the far-reaching connections between dietary habits and general health and well-being. My quest for the perfect diet has been a personal journey through every dietary fad and fashion of the last 20 years, and the answers I've come up with today have surprised me perhaps more than anyone else.

In the early 1970s, while I was spending my junior year in London and Israel, I became a vegetarian. I considered myself very socially aware with a strong spiritual consciousness and I believed it was very bad to eat meat and other animal products. I felt that fruits, vegetables, seeds, and nuts were man's natural foods and meat was not. I read as much as I could about vegetarian and raw food diets and all the evidence seemed to support my choices.

Natural hygiene, developed by Herbert Shelton, a version of which was later popularized in the best-selling diet book *Fit for Life* by Harvey and Marilyn Diamond, was one of the first guides that greatly influenced how and what I ate. My diet consisted primarily of raw fruits and vegetables, since the nutrition philosophy at that time was that cooking destroys enzymes, which in the 1970s were referred to as the "spark plug of life." I also drank a lot of green juice drinks made of leafy vegetables and ate a variety of nuts and seeds. I loved almonds, so they became my primary snack food; I had pockets full of them all the time. Carrot juice was my favorite between-meals pick-me-up. I was a walking example of a health nut!

In Israel and England, I met a lot of people following this diet who looked great. I lived with the family of a naturopathic physician who had followed a "living foods" diet for ten years; his children were strong and vital, and he and his wife both looked younger than their years. But, I did not do well on a vegetarian diet. My mind was dictating how healthy I was supposed to be by eating this way, but my body knew better. By the time I flew home from my experience abroad, I had lost a lot of weight and my hair, which had become weak and brittle, was cropped so short that the flight attendant called me "sir"! During my senior year in college, I realized how ill I was when my hair really started falling out and my skin kept breaking out. Instead of being the picture of health, I was wasting away. I thought I was getting sufficient amounts of protein through the nuts, seeds, and vegetables I was eating, but I was wrong. My parents, who were even more worried than I was about my health, finally took me to a physician, who told me my blood tests showed I had very low serum total protein and uric acid values. He said that I must start eating animal protein right away.

The bottom line is this: Although it seemed that a strict vegetarian diet worked for some people, it didn't work for me. In fact, it took at least a year and half after I finished college for my skin to finally clear up and a total of three years to regain my health after I started eating meat again. I still have the acne scars as a reminder of the severe imbalance I had imposed on my body. I worked hard at balancing my vegetarian diet then, but that wasn't enough. I know now that based on my biology—*my* unique metabolic rate, blood type, and ancestry—animal protein is a necessary component of *my* daily diet.

How James Influenced My Quest

Many years later I met James Templeton. James had cured himself of fourth-stage melanoma (skin cancer)with a strict macrobiotic diet, a fact that excited me and set me once again on the path of personal experimentation. (When I first met James, he was strictly macrobiotic but went on to eat fish later. I will discuss this change further on in this chapter.) On learning about the macrobiotic program from James, I liked certain ideas of the philosophy behind it: eating foods that were in season and that were available locally. I also liked some of the spiritual foundations of the plan, its holistic sense of balance and harmony in the universe, which had attracted me to vegetarianism as well. Macrobiotics is derived from the Greek words *macro,* which means "large" or "great," and *bio,* which means "life." It is a total way of life that embraces the concept of yin and yang, or expansion and contraction, and applies this concept to every aspect of life including the art and science of eating. I reasoned that if this diet could be traced to a documented cure for cancer, it seemed to me to be the perfect diet for everyone.

Once again, I learned the hard way. A macrobiotic diet is essentially a meatless diet and, although 20 years before my doctor had told me that I needed to eat meat, I was so motivated by the spirit of this eating plan that I decided to pursue macrobiotics in spite of the doctor's orders. I followed a macrobiotic diet for a year and, as with my previous vegetarian diet, I was very careful to plan it correctly. I ate miso soup and soft grains for breakfast; rice, beans, and sea vegetables for lunch, and dinners of more rice, soup, vegetables, and a tofu or fish dish. Soy sauce, vinegars, sesame seeds, and pickled foods were standard elements of the diet. Food preparation was complicated and time-consuming, and required a great deal of commitment and planning. Luckily for me, James liked to cook and was well versed in all the intricacies of macrobiotic cooking, so I knew we were doing it right.

Despite the fact that I was following the diet to the letter, my body didn't like the plan. I gained 10 pounds, felt sluggish midmorning and midday, and was constantly craving sweets. Although I was aware that the macrobiotic counselors were avid coffee consumers during those down times, I knew too much of the dangers of caffeine—the blood sugar highs and lows, the nerves on edge, and the inability to relax—to fall into that trap. I either went hungry or snacked on a never-ending supply of rice cakes, popcorn, and crackers. When I later reflected upon James's experiences at the Kushi Institute in Beckett, Massachusetts, the foremost center for macrobiotic studies in this country, I began to wonder about the rightness of a strict macrobiotic diet for me. Let me share a little about his health history and the initial success he had on this diet plan.

James's Quest for a Health-Supporting Diet

In 1985, at the age of 32, James seemed the picture of success. Caught up in the American dream in Huntsville, Texas, he was well on his way to making his first million dollars. Happily married and the proud father of an infant daughter, he was totally shocked when he was told he had fourth-stage melanoma. Even with the recommended surgery and chemotherapy, he was informed that his chance of survival was a mere 20 percent.

After the initial shock had worn off, James decided there had to be a way for him to fight his illness. He chose to forego the traditional cancer treatment route. Although he had been a meat-and-potatoes man from cattle country—Texas—he broke away from his old habits and began a self-healing journey that led him to Michio Kushi, one of the leaders of the macrobiotic movement in the United States. James studied with Kushi for two years and put his business acumen to work at the Kushi Foundation, acting as purchasing manager for the institute's educational center. During that time, with help from the inspirational messages of John Denver's music, James gained invaluable insights into the nature of his illness and, more importantly, the elements that contributed to his health.

But, after four years on a strict macrobiotic diet, blood tests and live blood cell analysis revealed that he had become very deficient in protein, vitamins, and certain nutrients, especially essential fatty acids. He was also tired much of the time and didn't have his former long-term endurance. This was not this once-energized Texan's idea of being fully cured!

The macrobiotic diet had been very helpful for him in the initial stages of his healing but, for the long haul, he realized he needed to expand the diet. His body was no longer in the healing stage but in the rebuilding stage. His cancer was in remission. He was starting to work and wanted to vigorously exercise again. To gain the protein and nutrients he was lacking, James added more fish, vitamin $B_{12,}$ and essential fats in the form of flaxseed oil to his diet. He also experimented with small amounts of organic beef in beef stew, which he ate once a week. As a result, James felt more energetic almost immediately. James also began to realize that while many individuals did remarkably well on the macrobiotic diet, there were those who did not.

With his new understanding of the importance of supplements to a balanced diet, James started a mail-order company called Uni-Key Health Systems, which specializes in unique nutrition products for the nineties. Many of the supplements that I recommend in this book are available through Uni-Key and were beneficial to his own healing. (The address and toll-free number are listed on page 190)

James and I met because he first became a client of mine. His initial success with the macrobiotic diet propelled me to try the plan and, when James offered to cook for me, I couldn't resist the tempting offer. Although it is said that food is the road to a man's heart, women will attest that it is the road to a woman's heart as well. Today James is my "significant other" and provides my clients and readers with supplements and books through Uni-Key.

Throughout all of this, James I both discovered some of the same principles of diet and nutrition. First of all, a diet that is designed to be therapeutic, like the macrobiotic diet and certain juicing diets, may not necessarily be effective on a long-term basis as a life-style or maintenance diet. Also, I have come to the undeniable conclusion—with James's help—that, in fact, there is no one diet that is perfect for everyone. The good news is, there is an individually perfect diet that is suitable for each one of us.

Breaking Away from Conventional Dietary Wisdom

This book represents another stage in my personal journey. If what you have been eating lately has been dictated by the magazines you read, the diet books on the bookstore shelves, and the infomercials on late-night television all proclaiming the new dietary wisdom of low fat and high carbohydrates, then this book is for you. If you have made choices about what to eat based on political agendas or if vegetarianism has become something of a religion to you, then I'm glad you're reading this. The truth is that we have to look at factors in our very biology, in our genes, that determine what we each should be eating. Each of our bodies holds the clues that tell us what we should eat. If we just know where to look for them, we can pinpoint what we need to do for ourselves.

The theory I propose is somewhat revolutionary in the nutrition field. Going against the grain has not been an easy task, but it is something I have had to do because so many are suffering from following the conventional dietary wisdom. In my professional observations, I have seen many, many people strictly adhering to a carefully measured low-fat diet with an abundance of complex carbohydrates and a minimum of meat products. Instead of feeling energetic and enjoying new, slender figures, they have become overweight and malnourished. They don't consume enough essential fats to support weight loss, hormonal balance, or steady nerves, so they suffer from PMS, short tempers, and mood swings. There is often insufficient protein in such a diet, which can lead to fatigue and lack of endurance. In addition, the constant consumption of breads, pastas, and other grain-based foods has plagued some of my clients with food allergies, candidiasis, bloating, blood sugar imbalance, and other symptoms. In some cases, the thyroid and adrenal glands, which are the all-important energy and stress glands, can go unsupported by this diet, leading to a lowered level of immune strength and a lowered resistance to emotional stress. In other words, these poor clients are a mess, even though they're following their diet plan to a T.

Certainly with my work at the Pritikin Longevity Center, I saw many individuals who thrived on a diet that cut out fat and increased the carbohydrate intake. People who had heart problems and diabetes especially benefited from the reduced intake of fat in their diet. My own father, an adult-onset diabetic, was able to lower his consistently high blood sugar levels when his total fat intake was reduced, but he could only lower those levels to a certain point. It was only when he reduced the total amount of carbohydrates he consumed in addition to the fat he consumed that he was able to completely normalize his blood sugar levels.

The key for him was to increase his intake of lean protein, not complex carbohydrates.

The popular belief that this one diet (low fat, high fiber, high complex carbohydrate) is the solution to *all* of our health concerns has turned out to be a myth. It sells magazines, that's for sure. And it's sold us on pasta as a gourmet meal. As you will learn, there are some people who do very well on this particular diet, but by no means is it sufficient for large numbers of our population. This particular diet is especially problematic for people like myself and my clients who either burn off carbohydrates too quickly or not quickly enough. Both the *fast burners* and the *slow burners* have a metabolic rate that's just a little faster or slower than normal, and, therefore, both struggle with weight gain and other unhealthy symptoms.

If recent statistics are any indication, it appears, in fact, that the low-fat, high-carbohydrate diet has backfired for the majority of Americans. The latest results from a long-term study by the Centers for Disease Control and Prevention show that the percentage of overweight Americans has increased from one quarter of the population in 1980 to one third of the population in 1990. That's a 30 percent increase, the most alarming escalation in overweight Americans in just a single decade! Even though many Americans with the best of intentions are following today's conventional dietary wisdom, they are fatter than they ever have been and are suffering from all the health problems that accompany weight gain.

Resurrecting Overlooked Dietary Factors

So, if this one diet won't work, what does one do? How does one know what diet is healthy and works? That is the very question James and I asked ourselves. To answer it, I put together all of the clues James and I had been collecting through our years of research and experience. Once I could find the common threads among the different schools of thought on the matter of nutrition, I was sure I could find a way to roll them into an easy-to-follow plan with something for everyone. My goal is that each and every individual who wants to lose weight and enjoy optimum immunity from disease and quality longevity will be able to benefit from our research and experiences that we share now.

In this book, I present information that refutes the current dietary wisdom about the benefits everyone can gain from an extremely low fat, extremely high carbohydrate diet. There are some fundamental facts about protein, fat, and carbohydrates that even the experts have overlooked or ignored in their quest for the perfect diet. In fact, if you don't have a clear understanding of the way each of these nutrients work, you could be setting yourself up for a weight-loss diet that not only fails but could jeopardize your health as well.

You will read about:

- how some people actually need both protein and the right kind of fat in order to lose weight
- two hormones—insulin and glucagon—that play an enormous role in the storage of body fat and the accumulation of unwanted pounds
- how excessive consumption of fruit and fruit juices can actually make you fat
- the dangers, including weight gain and food allergies, of overloading your system with wheat and dairy products
- innovative new information that implicates hydrogenated products like margarine and vegetable shortening with their high trans fatty acid content in the epidemic of heart disease and cancer
- anthropological proof that the human body is designed for a diet based on animal products

I'll focus on the idea that *different people require different diets,* that following a diet suitable for your unique biological needs is what nature intended in the first place. I've also put together a primer on the true role of carbohydrates, fats, and proteins in the body so you will no longer be afraid to eat the very foods your body needs. My research will give you permission to eat many of the foods that have for so long been forbidden.

When we put it all together, you'll be able to determine, based on your own body, which foods are best for you to eat and which are best to avoid. I'll run through some currently popular diets with a brief explanation of how they're supposed to work and why they work for some people but not for others. You might be surprised how much of mother's wisdom is part of my recommendations: eat balanced meals, get outside in the sunshine, and exercise.

Food for Thought

If you have been following some version of the low-fat, high-carbohydrate diet that's been all the rage for the last several years, why are you still overweight? Is it you, or is it the diet?

If all these popular diets are supposed to make you feel healthy as well as slim, why don't you feel better? Where's all the energy this high-carbo regime is supposed to provide?

How many days in a row have you sat down to three well-balanced meals? Do we even know what well-balanced means these days?

Have you looked at the weight patterns of your parents and siblings lately? How many times have you watched family members agonize over diet?

YOUR
BODY
KNOWS
BEST

1

Why Different People Require Different Diets

Betsy is your typical high-powered Chicago executive. She walks fast, talks fast, and thinks even faster. You might say she's always on the fast track. Betsy, 35, keeps up with all the latest nutrition information and, therefore, has cut out all fats from her diet and has increased her intake of fiber-rich grains, breads, pasta, and potatoes as the current diet plans dictate. She keeps a diet soda on her desk at all times and, after a hard day at work, treats herself with fat-free yogurt (which tastes even sweeter than ice cream, thanks to the miracle of NutraSweet). Believing that she can "eat more, weigh less," Betsy cannot understand why she is not losing but gaining weight, is tired all the time, and feels uncomfortably bloated in her abdominal area. Knowing that her diet couldn't be the culprit, Betsy has increased her exercise program. When that doesn't help, she becomes convinced that she suffers from chronic fatigue syndrome. Her blood type is B and her grandparents come from Eastern Europe.

1

Monica is a real fitness fanatic. At the age of 42, she is a competitive cyclist in Boston who looks exceedingly fit and has only an 8 percent body fat level. Unfortunately, she doesn't feel healthy. A family history of elevated cholesterol levels has made her a strict convert to the low-fat, high complex-carbohydrate propaganda, and she has cut all meat and animal products from her diet. But after three years on this regimen, she has begun to suffer from ongoing yeast infections, dry skin, dandruff, chest pains, and, finally, hair loss. Monica is of Irish ancestry, and has type O blood.

Now meet Linda, a 25-year-old hairdresser in Tucson. Linda has become a missionary for vegetarianism, and for good reason. Since giving up all animal products, including meat, chicken, fish, and dairy, she feels lighter and more energetic and has lost 20 pounds. She has no more digestive upsets and can finally jump out of bed in the morning with vigor and vitality. Linda has type A blood; her ancestors hail from the Mediterranean area.

These three women, created as composites from the 7,000-plus case histories I've collected throughout my career as a nutritionist, are all following basically the same low-fat, high-carbohydrate diet, but with vastly different results. Monica experiences some pretty serious health problems; Betsy has been gaining weight; Linda has been so successful that she tries to get everyone she meets to try her extreme version of the diet. I've included the information about their blood types and ancestry for a very important reason: to illustrate that certain biological clues point the way to the kind of dietary information that we need. Why would all of these women on the same diet experience such different results? The reason is that each of their individual chemistries reacts differently to the diet.

Imagine an Eskimo on a low-fat diet. The traditional diet of Eskimos consisted of up to 10 pounds of meat a day, including high quantities of fat, but there is no evidence of cancer or heart disease in their history. Is it possible that through hundreds of generations, the Eskimos actually evolved genetically so their bodies *require* a diet high in protein and fat in order to stay healthy in their frigid environment? Now think about the typical Oriental or Indian diet, which has historically centered around vegetables and rice. Would this low-fat, low-protein diet provide enough stamina, endurance, energy, and body fat to withstand the extreme environment of the North Pole? Common sense would lead you to answer "No" and that, as it turns out, is the correct answer.

Personalized Nutrition—Not a New Concept

There is no universal diet suitable for everybody. It may seem like a new idea to you, but in fact, the concept of biological uniqueness and personalized nutrition has been around for centuries. Here's a little bit of international history to prove my point: Ancient Chinese writings and early Egyptian and Greek physicians all incorporated this concept into their healing dietary regimens. Hippocrates, often considered the father of medicine, classified individuals in different categories according to characteristics of their blood and phlegm and the color of the bile. Body structure was another feature Hippocrates told his students to observe when making diagnoses.

Traditional Chinese medicine has developed its own unique system of classifying disease symptoms individualistically. Using tools such as tongue, pulse, and deficiency or excess, yin or yang, and cold or hot patterns diagnosis, Oriental medicine practitioners choose a course of treatment and food therapy for each patient based on the results of their findings in these areas. Some foods and herbs are very strongly indicated and helpful for some individuals but are wrong for others who have different types of ailments. This personalized form of medicine, which was developed thousands of years ago, is still in use today and recently has been gaining renewed popularity in the United States.

Ayurveda is the 6,000-year-old science of India that differentiates individuals in reference to body typing. Color and texture of hair and skin, rate of speech, body size and shape, gait, and even temperament and emotional responses are the clues Ayurvedic physicians look at to determine body type, and assist them in individualizing diagnoses and treatment. Dr. Stuart Rothenberg, national co-director of the U.S. Maharishi Ayur-Veda Medical Center, explains it best. "Western medicine asks what kind of disease the patient is suffering from. Ayurveda asks what kind of patient is suffering from the disease."

Lucretius, the Roman philosopher, is credited with saying, "One man's meat is another man's poison." The fact is that the concept of nutritional individuality has been a recognized ingredient of good health since antiquity. In modern times as well, there have been many noted researchers who acknowledged the importance of personalizing health and nutrition. Henry Bieler, in his book *Food Is Your Best Medicine* (Random House, 1965), led the way in modern times with his classification of individuals according to the dominance of their adrenal, thyroid, or pituitary glands. Even before Bieler, body structure classifications were identified by Dr. William H. Sheldon in *The Atlas of Men* in the 1940s. He divided individuals into three basic types: ectomorph (thin), endomorph (fleshy), and mesomorph (muscular).

Perhaps the most well-known of these personalized health subscribers was the noted biochemist Dr. Roger Williams. He promoted his ideas of biochemical individuality as early as the 1950s, further explaining them in an interview in 1977: "(Biochemical individuality) simply tells us that body chemistries are not the same. Two people of about the same height and weight have about the same total metabolism, but the details of chemical reactions taking place in their bodies may be different. Certain reactions will take place ten times as fast in one individual as another. This makes our nutritional needs different."

Dr. William Donald Kelley systematized metabolic typing analysis with computer technology in the 1960s. He was also one of the early medical proponents of treating the patient based on his or her metabolic type rather than attempting to treat the disease. More recently, two-time Nobel Laureate Dr. Linus Pauling, in his extensive studies of the effects of vitamin C on health, confirmed the principle of biochemical individuality when he discovered that different people required different amounts of the nutrient for optimal nutritional health. For some people, the desired amount of vitamin C to be added to the daily diet (up to 10 grams) far exceeded the Recommended Daily Allowance (RDA) of 60 milligrams.

We are just beginning to understand the tremendous variation in individual nutrient needs and other aspects of biochemical individuality. I am certain that with more research in this area, we will find other factors in our genetic blueprint that affect our health. For example, veteran nutritional researcher Lendon H. Smith, M.D., has observed that blue-eyed blonds, green-eyed redheads, and American Indians develop alcoholism more frequently than other Americans. Perhaps there is something in their genes that make these groups more prone to contracting the disease.

Until more research is done, however, we need to look at what we do know about biochemical individuality. The place to start is with ancestry and heredity—that fascinating collection of unique biological factors that has developed in a group of people over hundreds of thousands of years of evolution. We have each inherited a distinctive set of nutritional needs based upon the effects of climate, geography and the indigenous foods of our ancestors. Whole cultures have genetically adapted over dozens of generations to various conditions and their bodies have developed an affinity and dependence upon the specific foods natural to their region. What is most surprising about this fundamental concept of biochemical individuality is that it has been virtually ignored by modern-day nutritionists, who have singularly focused their attention on creating one universal diet without any regard for genetic makeup.

Let's examine the ancestral diet a bit deeper, so you understand its significance as a key modifying factor in your personalized diet plan.

How Ancestry Influences Our Health

Most of us come from families that have been in this country for several generations, which may make our own genetic nutritional requirements seem less obvious than the examples of the traditional Eskimo and Oriental diets. Furthermore, few of us have a one-nationality lineage, making our genetic influences even more convoluted. In our frenzy to find one perfect diet, we've forgotten a basic tenet of our American heritage: The United States is a "melting pot."

While few of us, like the Native Americans, have descended from peoples who have been on the North American continent for dozens of centuries, vast numbers of us have come from other continents and may have lost touch with our cultural—and physical—origins. Most of us, in fact, have been here only for a few generations. Our parents, grandparents, or great-grandparents hail from Northern, Southern, and Eastern Europe, South America, Africa, and Asia. Some of us have come from harsh, unrelenting climates where fresh fruits and vegetables were rare and meat or heavy, cold-water fish were eaten several times a day. Others have ancestors who lived in tropical climates where fruits, fish, and grains made up the bulk of the daily diet. Some of us have learned to harbor our personal resources, slowing down our metabolism to build body fat to keep us warm in cold climates or when food is scarce. Others, who perhaps adjusted to several generations in a warm climate, grew to depend on a diet high in leafy vegetables, fruits, legumes, and fish and seldom ate fatty animal meats.

Taking Ancestry with Us

Remember, it's only been in the last few hundred years that humans have become as transitory as we are now, moving from one continent to another with ease. If we know where our ancestors are from, we're fairly safe in assuming that several generations remained in the same region back then. Through countless generations, then, our ancestors naturally adapted and biochemically adjusted to become perfectly suited to their own environment and the foods naturally available there. However, researchers have noted that ethnic and genetic conditions persist, even if people have moved from their original geographic location. That means that even though somewhere along the line your ancestors moved, they took the genetic and nutritional needs that they built at their original location with them. The key to where our ancestors came from and the kind of biochemical adjustments their bodies made is now in our own genes: they determine our highly individualized nutritional requirements, no matter where we live. Simply put, if we know our ancestry, we will have a much better idea of what might be the right foods for us to eat.

To prove my point, let's look at the work of Weston A. Price, D.D.S. Price, a pioneer in medical/nutritional anthropological research, traveled over 100,000 miles to over a dozen indigenous communities around the globe in the early 1930s. He looked at the diets and health of primitive and indigenous tribes in South America, Australia, Africa, Polynesia, and North America (Native Americans and Eskimos)—cultures that were beginning to experience the impact of modern civilization.

Carefully documenting the information he discovered about each population during his 20 years of research, Dr. Price concluded that the best diet for each of the populations he encountered is the diet of their own ancestors. Price's work showed that even though native diets were radically different from one location to the next, all the people within each tribe were able to maintain a standard of good health *until* they began eating foods not native to their own culture, such as processed carbohydrates like white sugar, white flour, and polished rice.

Price's book, *Nutrition and Physical Degeneration* (Price-Pottenger Foundation, 1945), is a real nutrition classic that is just as relevant today as it was when it was first published, not only for its emphasis on ancestral diets but also for the proof that it holds on the havoc that the so-called "civilized" foods (like white flour and white sugar) cause when they are introduced into native diets. Price determined that the native diets differed according to climate, geography, and the natural flora and fauna of the region, but the common factors of all these primitive tribes was that they each had evolved to eat the foods naturally available in their region: fresh vegetables and fruits, whole grains, nuts, and animal protein. My research has led me to this same conclusion.

Native Diets Nourish Best

Other researchers have found that when people stray from their indigenous diets, they miss out on the necessary nutrients that had been provided by their native diets. Certain groups of people have greater needs for different nutrients than others. For example, the Scottish, Welsh, Celtic, Irish, Danish, Scandinavian, and northern coastal Indian peoples all display an inherited need for more essential fats in their diet than other populations. People with this ancestry have bodies that are accustomed to a native diet high in fatty fish. While key nutrients of this kind of fatty fish are sorely lacking in most contemporary diets, they can be easily replaced in the diet when people of these ancestries eat foods that are similar to those in their own native diets. If they don't get these nutrients their bodies crave, they can suffer from disastrous consequences like alcohol abuse, anxiety, depression, and schizophrenia.

One group of contemporary researchers working with the concept of ancestral diet is an organization in Arizona called Native Seeds/SEARCH. The researchers in this organization have focused their attention on the Pima Indians in Tucson, Arizona. Based on their findings, the researchers' recommendations for the native tribe include turning away from the modern diet and returning to the original diet of their ancestors as a way to combat many illnesses, including adult-onset diabetes, which Pima Indians experience at the highest rate in the world. Their native foods, such as beans, chia seeds, psyllium seed, nopalitos, cholla buds, bellotas (Emory oak acorns), mesquite pods, and cactus are high in soluble fibers and naturally help regulate blood sugar. Since these foods have become less important in the modern diet, the health of the Pima Indians has suffered.

Native Hawaiians are another population that have experienced serious health problems in the years that their culture has turned away from their native diet. In fact, native Hawaiians now have the worst health profile in America. Death rates from obesity, cancer, heart disease, and diabetes are among the highest in the nation. Some doctors treating native Hawaiians are now prescribing a diet rich in native foods that include taro root, seaweed, sweet potatoes, greens, fruit, and small amounts of fish. Those who have followed a diet based on their native one have had extremely promising results.

Just How Different Are We?

A red flag of common sense should fly up in front of our eyes when we read specific dietary guidelines, whether they are vitamin and mineral Recommended Daily Allowances (RDAs) or the optimum number of calories and fat grams a person should consume. Think about it for a moment: Just how much alike in physical energy, body mass, bone structure, temperament, shape, and size are you when compared to just about anybody else? Aside from having the requisite number of internal organs in pretty much the standard places, wouldn't you agree that you are probably quite different from the next person?

Marion Patricia Connolly, director of the Price-Pottenger Nutrition Foundation, which was formed to promote the findings of nutritional pioneers Dr. Weston Price and Francis M. Pottenger, M.D., writes the following: "It all boils down to our genetic inheritance from the survival of the fittest, whether we are of Mediterranean descent or of Norwegian descent. . . . The former could handle grains, legumes and foods of the Mediterranean basin while the latter would do better with a high-mineral diet from the sea, tubers and the foods available during the 8,000 additional years when the home of their ancestors was limited in food production by the Wurm glaciation [the Ice Age]."

Changing from a diet natural to a person's physical heritage and environment to something "foreign" could spell trouble for that person's health, no matter how "healthy" the new diet seems to be for others. Much research to support the current low-fat, high-carbohydrate diet was actually done in indigenous cultures whose natural surroundings supported that sort of diet. There doesn't seem to be any direct proof, however, that a diet that is suitable for an aged population in Ecuador would necessarily work for a young person in America.

According to Nathan Pritikin, the pioneer of the extremely low-fat diet, many of our current dietary woes are due to certain elements in our diet that other cultures do not have. Among others, he researched the Bantus in Africa, whose diet is 10 percent fat and coronary heart disease is close to nil. Natives of New Guinea have a diet of 10 percent fat and only 7 percent protein;

out of 600 deaths, only 1 was attributable to coronary heart disease. Pritikin also refers to studies on an aged population in Ecuador whose diet is mainly complex carbohydrates: corn, brown rice, beans, and various other vegetables and fruits, with a once-weekly portion of animal protein. The Tarahumara Indians of northwestern Mexico's Sierra Madre mountains are famed for their high endurance levels and their wooden kickball races. These Olympic-caliber athletes subsist on a diet of 10 percent protein, 10 percent fat, and 80 percent complex carbohydrates, a diet that is tailor-made for their extraordinarily active life-style.

Dietary Transplants

Unfortunately, statistics such as these have compelled many diet gurus to transplant diets from other societies and other climatic regions into our society. While a typical Tarahumara may indeed have amazing strength, resiliency, and endurance on his diet for his highly physical life-style in which he burns tremendous amounts of carbohydrates, could his diet support an average overworked stockbroker of Irish descent working on Wall Street? The Bantus of Africa may do well on their 10 percent fat diet in Africa, but could a German–American sitting at a computer all day in Silicon Valley eat the same foods and thrive? And how would a 200-pound construction worker from Norway fare on the typical Ecuadorian diet?

These are the sorts of questions that have never before seemed important to consider. So much research has pointed to indigenous cultures and their health that we've rarely considered the other side of the coin. We imagine that if that diet worked for them in their native lands, it will work for us in our highly industrialized modern world. What's been missing is the idea that even busy, urbanized Americans have their own native diet based upon their own individual ancestry. We've been easily misled by the virtues of diets that work for other peoples in other places, and have tried to transpose them to our own society without any regard to our own personal history.

Analyzing Our Unique History

The answer, instead, is to look at our own individual ancestral diet. Although we may think of certain popular American foods, like hamburgers and apple pie, as part of our natural diet, the answer to a healthy diet for each of us lies a bit further back in our history. We need to look at the foods of our ancestors, in their native lands, because like the Eskimos and the Pima Indians, we are more genetically adapted to the foods once growing in abundance in the regions of our roots.

The traditional Mediterranean diet of fish, olive oil, garlic, beans, and pasta could suit those of us with Italian, Greek, and Spanish ancestry well. An Asian-American can still do well on a diet of brown rice, sea vegetables, tofu, and other soy products. Descendants of families from south of the border can still benefit from a diet rich in seafood, tropical fruits, beans, corn, and vegetables. Those of us descended from the original inhabitants of the Americas—Native Americans—would be wise to include our own ancestral foods as well, whether they are beans, squash, cactus, or buffalo. As Lendon H. Smith, M.D., wrote in *Happiness Is a Healthy Life:* "The trick of eating is to figure out your racial/ethnic background and try to imitate it."

But how many of us can say we are direct descendants from a specific tribe or race? Most of us have a little of this and a little of that. We're African-Hispanic. Irish-Italian. German-Russian. French-Venezuelan. Italian-Arabic. Swedish-Lebanese. Mixed ancestry does not have to cause a problem when you are trying to determine the best diet for you. Some of you will find that you tend more toward one nationality in your background than the others, just based on your physical characteristics and food tastes. Or, you might have the best of both worlds and be able to tolerate a wide variety of foods because of your vast genetic inheritance. All it takes is spending a little time paying attention to your own body and maybe doing a little family research.

Ancestry: A Quick Recap

- Knowing where our own family ancestors are from can provide clues about how our own family members naturally adapted and biochemically evolved to become suited to their own environment and the foods naturally available there.
- Researchers state that genetic and ethnic conditions persist even if people have moved from their original geographic location. That means that our nutritional needs are determined far more by where our ancestors originated than by where we live now.
- When people stray from their indigenous diets, they can miss out on specific and necessary nutrients and suffer from a host of physical and emotional difficulties.
- Basing our diets on the indigenous diets of other peoples can spell trouble, even when those diets appear to provide health and fitness. Incorporating those diets into our own lives doesn't take into account our own indigenous foods and special biochemical needs that have evolved over many generations.
- Most of us in North America are the product of generations of mixed ancestry, making strict determinations about a diet based solely on ancestral heritage very difficult. That's why we will consider several other components of the individual diet and view the ancestral nutritional needs as a modifying factor. Ancestry is not the only key to discovering the right diet for each of us. It's just one modifying factor among others, as I'll now explain.

How Our Metabolic Rate Influences Our Health

Even people in the same family experience differences in the way they process food and their dietary requirements. Robin eats like a horse and never seems to gain a pound, although she still complains of feeling fat. She goes to bed late, gets up early, and is never short of energy. Robin is often called high-strung by her more mellow siblings; she flies off the handle easily but her temper tantrums are brief. Her sister Carolyn, on the other hand, feels like she gains weight just by looking at food. Carolyn's temperament is much smoother than her sister's, but she also seems to move a lot slower. She's more methodical and laid back and is not easily upset except over her seeming inability to lose weight, no matter how careful she is about her diet.

Even though these women have the same ancestral background, their metabolism—how quickly their systems burn off fuel—is different. Could one diet possibly work for both sisters? Robin is so wound up, it probably wouldn't hurt to slow her down a little, but Carolyn could use an energy boost.

Imagine for a moment that their parents came from two very different ancestral backgrounds. Their mother's family was Northern European; her ancestors lived for many generations in a cold, harsh, and damp climate where few crops grew and the people relied heavily on a few sturdy root vegetables, breads, and meat. Their father's family, on the other hand, had been in the Mediterranean region for centuries; their diet was one of fruits, leafy vegetables, fish, grains, and legumes. It's easy to see how their offspring could have incorporated a whole range of influences, with some of their dietary needs reflecting their mother's heritage and others reflecting their father's. But let's look beyond ancestry for a moment. Instead, let's look at what we saw in Robin and Carolyn in terms of the speed at which they burn up food for energy. These two sisters have two different **metabolic rates.**

Probably the most important and overlooked aspect in determining a person's bio-individuality is the rate at which a person turns his or her fuel into energy. Thanks to the insights of metabolic expert Bill Wolcott of HealthExcel (see the Appendix for a description of his organization), I was able to uncover this major clue to personalizing diet. The food we eat, along with water, air, and light, is used to maintain and sustain life on a minute-to-minute basis every day of our lives. The biochemical processes that use all of these components collectively are known as metabolism. The metabolic activity in which cells transform food into energy is called oxidation.

Like the engine of an automobile, your body needs the right kind of fuel to work properly and efficiently. If you know what will happen if you put diesel fuel (or water) into your gasoline engine, you can imagine the negative consequences of eating food that your system just isn't designed to handle.

Slow Burners and Fast Burners

Dr. George Watson, Ph.D., of the University of Southern California, first connected the oxidation rate with metabolic individuality in the 1970s. As a psychologist, Watson was primarily concerned about the effects of oxidation rate on the emotions and behavior of his patients. He identified two types of oxidizers who do not use energy efficiently: the slow oxidizer and the fast oxidizer, which I have already referred to as the **slow burner** and the **fast burner**. Other researchers, such as Drs. Paul Eck, Dave Watts, and Rick Malter, have all expanded our knowledge about the oxidation types and their effect on dietary needs and psychological problems.

Both oxidation types can experience problems with their weight. Robin is a fast burner, and her sister Carolyn is a slow burner. As you might have guessed, these two terms refer to the relative speed at which a person is able to utilize nutrients—like carbohydrates, proteins, and fats—for energy. Although you might be tempted to think that if you have problems keeping extra weight off then you are a slow burner, that's not the case at all. Fast burners, especially if they don't eat the right foods for their metabolism, can have just as much trouble trying to budge those extra pounds.

You see, energy is created by the interaction of two biochemical processes in the body—glycolysis and the citric acid (or Krebs) cycle. Simply speaking, these processes require very specific minerals and vitamins at every stage of energy production. Both the slow and fast burners, due to their own specific set of vitamin and mineral deficiencies, do not utilize energy efficiently. The slow burner burns food too slowly, and therefore can feel lethargic and sluggish and gain weight easily. The fast burner burns food too quickly, especially carbohydrates, and so can feel hyped up, nervous, and easily stressed. Fast burners also burn out quickly, stripping them of the energy needed for exercising, the lack of which contributes to weight gain.

Slow burners tend to gravitate toward simple carbohydrates such as sodas, candies, pastries, and other sugary foods in a misguided attempt to create quick energy. Long-lasting energy is created much more readily with moderate amounts of lean protein that could be missing from a slow burner's diet. A slow burner is much better off satisfying her sweet tooth with small amounts of fruit or sweet vegetables like butternut squash or yams, rather than sugary snacks, however, because of the uneven blood sugar swings the sugary snacks cause.

Oftentimes, a glucose tolerance test, which tests for the ability to metabolize sugars, reveals high blood sugar or diabetes in slow burners. Slow burners also tend to have a higher than normal insulin level (hyperinsulinemia), which results in conversion of carbohydrates into body fat. (I'll be explaining the insulin connection to carbohydrates and body fat in more detail in the next chapter.) Another characteristic of slow burners is that they generally have a poor appetite and dislike protein-rich foods and fats. A thick, juicy steak or rich, cheesy sauces are not very appealing to these types. Instead, they tend to overindulge in starches such as pasta and bread, which can lead to overeating and weight gain. Because a slow burner's energy production is slowed down, the efficiency of the glandular system can also be affected, particularly the thyroid and adrenal glands, which tend to be hypoactive—or underactive. This can lead to a sense of constant fatigue, exhaustion, apathy, and depression, and a sense of feeling cold all the time.

Fast burners, on the other hand, usually show a low blood sugar reading on a glucose tolerance test because their energy cycles are burning off carbohydrates at a rate that is too fast. They are often diagnosed as hypoglycemic, or having low blood sugar. In the fast burning system, carbohydrates are metabolized so quickly that they don't offer a source of sustained energy. Fast burners can be likened to a furnace with fast-burning fuel. Without sufficient fat and protein in the diet to balance things out, fast burners feel hyper and are often irritable and anxious. They, too, reach for more carbohydrates in the quest for a balanced blood sugar, but excessive carbohydrates only feed the flame of a fast burner. Try pouring gasoline on a fire if you want a clear picture of what carbohydrates do to the system of the fast burner. The blood sugar rises quickly, increasing the metabolic rate and all metabolic activity, causing a sense of nervousness or excitability. Next comes the crash as the blood sugar drops, following its quick removal from the blood. At this time, the fast burner is likely to feel fatigue and confusion as well as strong cravings for sugary foods. A constantly fluctuating blood sugar level—and the attendant mood swings—results. The remedy? A diet heavier in certain types of protein and **healthy** *fats* not only stabilizes blood sugar but also reduces cravings for sweets.

Fast burners also have strong appetites; they like to eat all the time. Heavy proteins like beef ribs or a plate of lamb chops satiate and sustain fast burners, giving them a sense of having been well-nourished. Although they appear filled with nervous energy, fast burners often keep themselves going with sheer will-power; their emotional state is often marked by extreme peaks and valleys and patience is not one of their strong suits. Fast burners can be overweight, just like slow burners, if they eat inappropriate foods for their metabolism. A diet heavy in processed and simple carbohydrates, such as pasta, fruit, and fruit juice, can lead to storage of body fat. I know the fast burner's pitfalls very well because I am one.

The common denominator for both types of fuel burners is that they need **protein** to stabilize their blood sugar levels. The fast burner needs heavier, fattier proteins such as red meat, organ meats, and cold-water fish daily. The slow burner, on the other hand, does not handle fat well (it slows down the metabolism) and so needs to eat lean protein, such as white-meat chicken, turkey, and fish, in the daily diet. I know that recommending a daily intake of forbidden foods such as steaks and ribs flies in the face of all the nutritional advice of the last several years. I myself have had a difficult time reconciling the fact that as a fast burner, I do feel significantly better following these guidelines of moderate meat intake than I did in my days as a vegetarian, macrobiotic, or Pritikin advocate. My body does well with these foods; it breaks then down and utilizes them for quality energy in a way it could not when I was on a high-carbohydrate diet.

You can see a magnified version of how important the distinction between the fast burner and the slow burner is by looking at children. Many children who are hyperactive or have attention-deficit disorder (ADD) are fast burners. With overactive adrenal and thyroid glands, they have trouble harnessing their nervous energy and are often irritable, aggressive, or even violent. Unfortunately, their parents, in a misguided effort to control cholesterol and fat, give these children all the wrong foods. Avoiding butter, meat, cheese, eggs, and other high-protein and fatty foods, the children fill up on cereal, bread, fruit, and other sweets. As I've explained, this sort of diet only aggravates the fast burner's already revved-up system.

Throughout my years of experience, I have seen very few balanced burners—people who fall into the normal range. Most people are either too fast or too slow, and many of them suffer from weight problems. In addition, a person's metabolic rate can be directly affected and in fact normalized by what he or she eats, which is why it is important for everyone to know if he or she is a slow or fast burner. If your metabolism is too slow, eating the right foods can speed it up. If it is too fast, the proper diet can actually slow it down. In either case, approaching a balanced rate of metabolism will result in achieving your desired weight and a healthier body, as well as smoothing out emotional ups and downs.

Diet Basics for Slow and Fast Burners

I'll go into much greater detail about the right diet for fast and slow burners in later chapters, but I want to give you a few standards to start with. As I mentioned, the best diet for a slow burner would be one that is low in fat, because fat slows down the already depressed metabolic rate. Processed and simple carbohydrates (sugar, honey, soft drinks, pasta, bagels, breads) should be eliminated or at least limited, due to the inherent problems slow burners have with blood sugar and insulin levels. Complex carbohydrates (winter squash, sweet potatoes, corn on the cob, peas) eaten with lean proteins will provide the slow burner with sustained energy. Protein will speed up the metabolic rate and therefore should be a consistent and daily part of the slow burner's diet. It should also be included because protein produces a hormone called glucagon, which blocks the fat-promoting activity of insulin, which is released when carbohydrates are eaten. Lean meats like chicken, turkey, and white fish will go a long way toward activating the metabolism of the slow burner. This is why certain individuals have had such outstanding success on diet programs like Weight Watchers, Diet Center, Lean Bodies, and Overeaters Anonymous. All these plans are actually geared to the person who is a slow burner. Slow burners also need more potassium, which can be found in citrus fruits and bananas, because it accelerates the metabolic rate.

By contrast, the fast burner would suffer on such low-fat diets. Fast burners do best on a diet that is higher in heavier protein and fat and low in complex carbohydrates. This diet helps to balance out blood sugar, create an enduring energy source, and also provide body warmth in cold weather. Roast beef, beef ribs, and lamb chops are necessary energy sources for the fast burner. This is a far cry from the diet of the slow burner, who thrives on lighter proteins like chicken and turkey. Fast burners also do well with foods that are high in calcium (such as broccoli, sesame seeds, and sea vegetables) because calcium tends to slow down the metabolic rate.

In addition, a certain class of proteins called nucleoproteins is very effective for the fast burner but should be avoided by the slow burner. Nucleoproteins provide substances called purines, which provide energy for the fast burner. (Fast burners do not produce this particular energy source in their own cells, whereas slow burners actually do.) Purine-rich proteins include wild game, red meats, anchovies, herring, caviar, sardines, and organ meats like liver, kidneys, sweetbreads, and heart. Although these may be unpopular foods today, they actually have been a standard meal component throughout our history. In fact, it has only been in the last 20 years when the misguided cholesterol propaganda came into vogue that these foods have been banished from the American home. Ancestrally speaking, organ meats were often considered to be the prize of a successful hunt. More recently, a quick scan of the most enduring cookbooks, such as *The Joy of*

Cooking, will reveal dozens of recipes for organ meats, high-lighting their presence in the American diet for decades.

The Atkins diet and other similar high-protein, high-fat diets may be most effective for the fast burner for weight loss and maintenance. This type of diet will reduce the craving for carbohydrates and sweets, and the relatively high fat content exerts a slowing effect on the fast burner's excessively fast rate of metabolism, resulting in improved energy efficiency. Dairy products can be beneficial for fast burners because they contain calcium, fat, and the amino acid tryptophan, which are all slowing agents. But one should also take into account an individual's personal level of tolerance for dairy products, by way of blood type and ancestral diet, before incorporating any number of them into a daily diet.

A complete discussion of the appropriate foods and sample menus for slow burners and fast burners can be found in Chapter 9.

Metabolism: A Quick Recap

- Probably one of the most important and overlooked aspects in determining a person's bio-individuality is the rate at which a person turns his or her fuel into energy.
- There are two types of people whose metabolisms do not burn energy efficiently; I call them the fast burner and the slow burner. Both can experience weight problems.
- Both fast and slow burners tend to eat diets high in carbohydrates, which contribute to weight gain. Slow burners burn food too slowly, can feel lethargic and sluggish, and gain weight easily. Fast burners use food energy up too quickly, and can feel hyped up, nervous, and easily stressed. Fat accumulates when the wrong foods are eaten and when the fast burner is too exhausted to exercise.
- Carbohydrates don't process quickly enough in the slow burner

and convert to fat; carbos also speed up the already speeding fast burner. Protein will jump-start the slow burner and also will provide more substance for the fast burner, balancing out the excessive highs and lows. Fat will slow down the slow burner and accumulate; the fast burner benefits from this slowing activity of dietary fat.

- Fast burners need more of the rich, red meats like beef, pork, and lamb, as well as dark meat poultry and cold-water fish. Fast burners also can eat more fat like full-fat dairy products to slow down their hyped-up metabolism.
- Slow burners do best with lighter forms of protein like white meat poultry and white fish. Slow burners can use more carbohydrates but not in the excessive amounts we've all become accustomed to in the last few years. Slow burners also need to be more watchful about fat intake in the form of dairy products and oils.

How Blood Type Influences Our Health

In addition to knowing where our ancestors came from and our rate of metabolism, there is another modifying factor that must be taken into account in personalizing a diet. Our own heritage is intimately tied in with blood type, a determination that evolved along with our other characteristics. The different blood types (A, B, AB, and O) appeared at different times during humankind's evolution and are related to the movement of generations of people over the continents. Although most of us are familiar with the standard ABO system of blood typing, few of us may realize how those different blood types connect us intimately to our distant past. Fewer still understand that our own blood type may be the secret clue to what the best foods are for each of us. Research also has indicated that blood type might affect our vulnerability to disease.

In Japan, the study of blood type and its impact on personality is serious business. Toshitaka Nomi has published over 25 books on the subject (including *You Are Your Blood Type*, Pocket Books, 1983) and is considered to be the world's foremost expert. Companies in Japan such as Honda, Toyota, and Yamaha frequently consult blood type information when determining consumer preference for marketing and manufacturing, or compatibilities among employees. Nomi also has postulated that national personality traits of Americans, Germans, and Japanese are based on the different balances between the blood type groups in their populations.

Nomi suggests that in general, blood type O's are goal oriented and enthusiastic, while blood type A's are more detail oriented and fastidious. Blood type B's tend to be creative and unconventional, whereas type AB's have a great spiritual sensitivity.

In North America, there have been two prominent naturopathic physicians, James D'Adamo and his son Peter D'Adamo, who have extensively researched blood groups in their relation to biochemistry, diet, and disease. You may want to refer to the published papers of Peter D'Adamo for more scientific documentation (see the References). In the book *The D'Adamo Diet* (McGraw-Hill, 1989), which is oriented more for the lay reader, James D'Adamo writes that because blood carries nutrients throughout the body, perhaps different blood types act differently with foods and their nutrient components. He found that people who had blood type A did well on a vegetarian or near-vegetarian diet, as did those with the very rare type AB, but individuals with type B need more animal protein in their diet. Type O's found it virtually impossible to remain on a vegetarian diet and feel healthy; as the oldest blood type, O's have been found to have a much greater genetic need for animal protein and fat. Type O's also tend to be much more physical, while A's are considerably less so, expending more of their energy in mental processes.

Before we look more closely at which foods are appropriate for the different blood types, let's examine the underpinnings of Dr. D'Adamo's findings. If it's true that different blood types react differently to different foods, then our next question might be, why do people have different blood types? The answer is one I've referred to several times: evolution. As humans moved across the planet in search of food, their bodies gradually adapted to whatever local conditions they found. (By gradually, of course, we mean over the course of millions of years. Evolution is such a slow process, a few generations are not sufficient to help the body adapt. That's one of the reasons why so many of us have trouble with sugar; it's only been available to us in its refined state and in abundance for the last 150 years!)

BLOOD TYPE O CHARACTERISTICS

Type O was the first blood type researchers have been able to determine existed among our ancestors. The very first humans were all type O and their diets reflected the first foods they found available. Animal meat (including fish) was their *primary* source of food, with roots, leaves, wild grains, and other foraged plant foods supplementing the meat. According to Dr. D'Adamo, type O's also have a high level of hydrochloric acid and other digestive enzymes, which make digesting a high-protein diet fairly easy. High levels of hydrochloric acid also make type O's less prone to developing parasitic infections like *Giardia*, yet they are actually more susceptible to infection by *H. pylori*, the bacteria that has been found to cause duodenal and peptic ulcers.

In humankind's earliest days, diary products cultivated from domesticated animals were unheard of, so the type O human did not completely adapt to be able to digest those foods. Some modern type O's might have a hard time with dairy products, finding them difficult to digest; they may produce gas and bloating, and may convert quickly into body fat.

More so than other blood types, type O's also have a greater predisposition to celiac/sprue disease, which is caused by a genetically inherited metabolic inability to digest foods that contain gluten, specifically, wheat, rye, oats, and barley. (Coincidentally, these grains are the "new foods" that were introduced into the human diet only 10,000 years ago, long after the first appearance of the type O person.) Symptoms of sprue include nausea and vomiting (especially in infants and children), severe flatulence, fatty stools, chronic constipation or diarrhea, bleeding from the colon, bloating and abdominal distention, fatigue and muscle weakness, memory loss, and depression. Hives, food allergies, and hay fever also are common among type O's.

Those early type O's were a very active sort; they needed to be in order to survive in a hunter/gatherer society. Today's type O's do well with a lot of vigorous exercise, like aerobics several times a week. Dr. D'Adamo suggests that type O's exercise frequently to increase energy and ward off fatigue and depression. In work with my clients, I've found exercise to be almost more important than eating correctly for those with type O blood.

BLOOD TYPE A CHARACTERISTICS

Type O was followed some centuries later by type A. Both blood types are now the most common in America, accounting for almost 85 percent of the population. Type A is predominant in Europe and Africa. Type A's tend to be "adaptive vegetarians," having developed when the wild meat supply dwindled and our ancestors turned to an agrarian life-style. Rather than a strict vegetarian diet for type A's, Dr. D'Adamo suggests incorporating fish, chicken, and turkey into the diet a few times a week. Red meat and dairy products are not recommended for this blood type because usually the A's stomach has a low output of hydrochloric acid and digestive enzymes.

To complicate matters, there are actually two type A's, called

A-1 and A-2. Most A-1's have lost the ability to make pepsin (a protein-digesting enzyme) but have other enzymes that aid in carbohydrate digestion. A-1's don't do too well with meat and dairy products, nor do they handle beans well. A-1's do best on a diet heavy in vegetables, fruits, nuts, seeds, and eggs. A-2's have more stomach acid and so can handle more meat and fish in the diet. Both types need to be careful about overdoing grains and concentrate on eating a broad variety of the foods just mentioned.

One of the reasons I found the research on blood types to be so fascinating is that while I was working on my book about intestinal parasites, *Guess What Came to Dinner*, I found that type A's are at high risk for infection by *Giardia*, a common waterborne parasite. It is the lack of hydrochloric acid in the digestive systems of most type A's that makes them so susceptible. Type A's also tend to have more digestive problems—gas, bloating, gastritis, and constipation—than the other blood types. Ulcers could be a problem for type A's because they seem to have more *Camphylobacter* bacteria in the digestive system. According to Dr. Peter D'Adamo, pernicious anemia and breast cancer can be more devastating for type A's because of certain immune responses in type A blood. Yeast overgrowth can also be a problem of type A's, and their immune systems tend to be somewhat sensitive, more good reasons for being aware of the proper diet for this types.

Type A's tend to be a lot less active than type O's; the blood type developed as humans began to utilize their minds for solving problems. Light exercise, such as stretching or occasional swims, are good for type A's, D'Adamo says, but they need to be careful of exhaustion, a tendency for type A's who are filled with nervous energy. Relaxation is important for blood type A's, who are sensitive and tend to get stressed out easily. Heavy exercise depletes the mental clarity of the type A.

BLOOD TYPE B CHARACTERISTICS

Blood type B appeared less than 10,000 years ago, which was after the introduction of domestic grains into the human diet. Type B's are predominantly of Eastern European and central Asian extraction, from societies that were nomadic herders. Natives of those areas are famous for their longevity, for which they wholeheartedly recommend yogurt. This is explained by the fact that type B's have digestive systems that are well adapted to dairy products, especially fermented ones like yogurt.

Type B also falls somewhere between type O and type A; thus, a person with type B blood can handle a range of animal products as well as a lot of complex carbohydrates. The key to the diet for type B's would be to find a good balance among different foods, as well as a balance between heavy or strenuous exercise and the more meditative types, such as yoga or t'ai chi. Type B's can also be more susceptible to degenerative conditions due to viruses.

BLOOD TYPE AB CHARACTERISTICS

Blood type AB, the rarest blood type, is perhaps the most well-adjusted for the new foods in our diet, such as dairy products and domesticated meats and grains. People with AB blood will generally lean more strongly to either the A type of energy level or the B, and can adopt either the A diet or the B diet (and level of exercise), depending on the individual. Meat, dairy products, and grain products may be tolerated less by AB's if they lean more toward having A characteristics, and those foods should be introduced slowly into the diet. If AB's lean toward having more B-type characteristics, they should be able to handle a wider range of foods. AB's may be more susceptible to chronic viral infections and cancer than the other types.

Currently, approximately 44 percent of the American Caucasian population have type O blood, as do 49 percent of American blacks. Blood type A is found in 42 percent of the white population, and only 27 percent of the black population. Only 10 percent of whites but 20 percent of blacks have blood type B, a more recently evolved type. Blood type AB occurs in only 4 percent of both groups in the American population. Discovering this information about blood types has been very exciting for me and, as I've studied D'Adamo's work, I've begun implementing many of his suggestions with my clients, with excellent results.

Another blood type determinant is the Rh, or Rhesus, factor. Most of us who have our blood tested know that we are either Rh negative or Rh positive. How that impacts on diet has yet to be investigated by blood type researchers, but you can bet I'll be following developments in this area in the future.

Blood Types: A Quick Recap

- Nutritional needs evolved along with the different blood types.
- Type O is the oldest blood type on the planet. Nutritionally, type O's adapted to a diet heavy in animal meat and fish on a daily basis, supplemented with roots, leaves, wild grains, and other foraged plant food. Type O's do not do well with dairy products or excessive amounts of grains, and they generally need to have active life-styles.
- Because of the lack of certain stomach acids that digest meat, type A's are best suited for a semivegetarian diet of leafy and starchy vegetables, incorporating the leaner meats like poultry several times a week but not necessarily every day. Type A's don't always handle dairy products very well, and should not overdo grains in the diet either. Type A's require less strenuous activity than type O's, and do best with light stretching and meditative exercises.
- Type B evolved with an ability to handle a wide variety of foods, and today should make an effort to find a balance between several different foods rather than focus on just a few.

• Type AB, the last to evolve, is very rare. It is the only blood type fully adapted to dairy products, but also may have some of the characteristics of an A type, which has less tolerance for meat and animal products.

Putting the Factors Together

I've covered three areas so far that will help you personalize your eating plan. Ancestry, metabolic rate, and blood type are three factors to consider when determining a diet that is appropriate for you. In my experience, the rate of metabolism should be the *dominant* factor when it comes to planning your diet, with blood type and ancestral heritage considered as *modifying* factors. For example, I am a fast burner with blood type B and an ancestral heritage that is Eastern European. As a blood type B, my diet can be fairly high in grain-based complex carbohydrates, but because my metabolism is so high, I do much better on a diet that is higher in protein and fats rather than carbohydrates. As an Eastern European with blood type B, I can also easily handle fermented dairy products like yogurt.

James, on the other hand, is a slow burner, with blood type O and ancestral heritage from northern Europe. As a blood type O, he needs more protein, but as a slow burner he needs to emphasize low-fat meats like chicken and fish rather than heavier meats like beef. Furthermore, as a northern European, he has a genetic need for high amounts of essential fatty acids, particularly those found in cold water fish like salmon.

Later on you'll learn about which foods are best for the fast burner and slow burner in greater detail, as well as for the different blood types and for people of different ancestral heritage so that you, too, can make a determination of the best diet for you. In the next chapter, I'll cover information that has been virtually ignored about carbohydrates and why certain types develop problems on the current popular high-carbohydrate diet.

Food for Thought

Take a look at yourself and then look at everyone else in your family, in your workplace, and in your circle of friends. You see many different shapes and sizes, different personalities and attitudes. How could one diet possibly be sufficient for all these different kinds of people? Now you know that the truth is, it can't be.

Take a moment to look at your family tree. What nationalities are your parents, and both sets of grandparents? Can you trace your roots back farther than that? Make some guesses about the foods that were eaten in the parts of the world your ancestors came from, and compare those foods to the foods you eat today, as well as the foods you most like or even crave.

Based on the outline of behavioral traits belonging to the different blood types, maybe you can make a guess at what your type is without having it tested. You can also look at the blood types of your parents and make some determinations about which traits or characteristics you may have.

Do you consider yourself high-strung and hyper, or are you more the slow and steady type? Do have a ravenous appetite that keeps you eating big meals several times a day, or do you find that one big meal fills you up for hours? Does the idea of a thick juicy steak seem like it would really satisfy you, or do you honestly crave a big salad instead? These are clues to whether you are a fast burner or slow burner, and to determine what you should be eating.

2

Carbohydrates:
The Optimum Fuel for
the Body?

Whether you actually follow them or not, if you're like millions of Americans, you can almost recite verbatim the dietary guidelines that have been espoused for at least the past decade by magazines, newspapers, diet books, and even the federal government: Cut the fat out of your diet. Eat more fruits, vegetables, and whole grains for fiber. Eat less red meat, or better yet, none at all, to lower your cholesterol level and avoid heart disease. Instead, eat more chicken (white meat, skinless) and fish, grilled or broiled but never fried. Eat more low-fat dairy products like yogurt for protein and calcium. Avoid sugar and fried snack foods. Instead, make carbohydrates the basis for your diet: cereal and toast for breakfast, pasta for dinner, rice cakes and fruit for snacks.

On the surface, the advice seems to make sense. If you eat less fat, you won't get fat. If you eat more complex carbohydrates (the body's preferred fuel source), like pasta and bread, you'll have more energy. If you eat more vegetables, your digestion will be smoother and easier. If you eat less cholesterol, you'll have a lower cholesterol level in your body.

It sounds easy, doesn't it? Maybe too easy. What a relief, you must have been thinking. I can eat more, weigh less, and stop the insanity of dieting! It's like the answer to all our dreams. Unfortunately, the high-carbohydrate/low- to no-fat diet has turned out to be a mixed blessing. It really is too good to be true. I have counseled many women who have not lost but have gained weight following this regimen to extremes. They eat massive amounts of potatoes, bread, and pasta; they eat very little meat; they've banished butter from their table and fat from their repertoire, and they fill up on "fat-free" yogurt, health food cookies, and gallons of no-fat fruit juice. *They have forgotten that weight gain can occur by eating too many calories not just by eating fat!*

Are they thin? No. Are they happy? No. They complain of fatigue, uncontrollable sugar cravings, irregular periods, and chronic yeast infections. When they cut back on all their carbohydrates (from pasta to fruit juice) and then reintroduce lean proteins (like fish, chicken, turkey, and even beef) as well as essential fats into their diets, their symptoms go away and their weight drops.

Latest Dietary Guidelines for Carbohydrates

In the new dietary guidelines espoused by the federal government (the Eating Right Food Pyramid, which has replaced the concept of the four major food groups), it is recommended that we each eat from 6 to 11 servings a day of complex carbohydrates, plus 3 to 5 servings of vegetables (which are also carbohydrates) and 2 to 4 servings of fruits (which are also carbohydrates).

Can anyone imagine eating that many plates of pasta? The idea, of course, is that you have toast and cereal for breakfast with fruit and fruit juice, a snack of a muffin before lunch, a sandwich and rice cakes or extra bread for lunch, and a snack of a bagel in the afternoon. Dinner consists of pasta or meat with a side dish of rice or potato, plus bread. Before bed, perhaps a piece of fruit. (That's not counting two to three servings a day of meat, fish, and eggs.) Aside from the fact that it seems like an awful lot of food for the average person to eat, what do all those carbohydrates do to the body? Before we take a new view of what carbohydrates are and how they work—fundamental biochemistry that unfortunately has often been overlooked—we should take a moment to understand the place carbohydrates hold in our history.

Historical Clues to the Role of Carbos

It is important to realize that domesticated grains and their refined products like flour, bread, and pasta are a very new addition to the human diet. Even white sugar, a refined food made from the sugarcane plant, has been around for only about 150 years! Although the 10,000 years since agriculture was first introduced seems like a long time to us, in the scope of human evolution, it is but a moment in time. As strange as it may seem, genetically, we have changed very little since the modern human being appeared 40,000 years ago. For the most part, our bodies are still Stone Age models.

Because only a few thousand years have passed since agriculture has come to play a part in our development, the human body has not had much of a chance to evolve or adapt to the new foods—grains and foods made from grains. In fact, it takes tens of thousands of years for even minor changes to occur, and hundreds of thousands or even millions of years for more significant changes. While some individuals seem to thrive on a largely grain-based diet, a significant portion of our population does not, simply because their bodies have not evolved enough to handle these foods. People who are sensitive to grains can suffer from malabsorption of nutrients, anemia, fatigue, and uncomfortable abdominal bloating several hours after eating. While most of us may have a genetic inability to handle these new foods—the grains—the excessive use of them is magnifying our problems with them. We're told they're the perfect food for the body, therefore, the more carbohydrates you eat, the more perfect you are. I disagree.

Carbos—Not for Everyone

The key is not to eat all the carbos in sight, but to know which foods work best for *you*, based on your own body type—your metabolic rate, your ancestry and heredity, and your blood type. As I have pointed out, our external differences like the color of our skin, the color of our eyes, the color of our hair, and even our personality are matched by our unique internal needs for different nutrients. Biochemical individuality is the most important factor to take into account when planning the right diet for yourself. Simply put, each person is able to handle a different amount of carbohydrates, as well as other nutritional building blocks, like protein and fats. There is no universal quantity or formula that applies to all of us.

What is the story with carbohydrates? Regardless of ancestry and body types, there are certain biochemical reactions that occur in the body when carbohydrates are eaten. Carbohydrates are energy foods; they are, in fact, the most preferred source of energy for the body. As a fuel, they are the cleanest burning. Carbohydrates provide glucose, which is necessary fuel for the brain, promoting clear thinking, level moods, and even, steady behavior patterns.

Carbohydrates also provide ready energy, which is especially important for the physically active. Without energy from some carbohydrates, the body will draw from the protein in its muscles for energy, resulting in a loss of muscle tissue and lean body mass.

It's no accident that the diet of choice for hard-working athletes is a diet with an emphasis on carbohydrates. However, as you will see in just a moment, even the long-considered truism of a high-carbohydrate diet for athletes is now being challenged by studies that show athletes receive significant performance benefits from a diet balanced between carbohydrates, protein, and fat, rather than one full of carbohydrates.

Although carbohydrates have been promoted as the miracle fuel for weight loss and as a high-energy food that won't make you fat, what most people don't realize is that the most commonly consumed carbohydrates (like pasta, bread, bagels, and potatoes) actually quickly release sugar into the bloodstream and then—if not immediately used—this sugar is turned into body fat! The body has only a limited amount of storage space for excess carbohydrates. It has, however, a limitless ability to turn excess carbohydrates into fat.

Simple Carbohydrates: Sugar and the Insulin Connection

As you may know, there are two kinds of carbohydrates, simple and complex. Simple carbohydrates are the sugars: mainly **table sugar** and **natural sweeteners** (like brown sugar, honey, molasses, corn syrup, and barley malt), **fructose** (which occurs in fruits and fruit juices and is also used as a natural sweetener), and **lactose** (found in dairy products like milk, cheese, ice cream, and yogurt). Complex carbohydrates are found in **starches** (whole grains and starchy vegetables like potatoes), **legumes** (beans and peas), and **vegetables** (like broccoli, asparagus, cabbage, carrots, and turnips).

Carbohydrates are energy foods, and simple carbohydrates provide more instant energy than the more long-lasting complex carbohydrates. When simple sugars and highly processed carbohydrates are eaten, they are broken down almost immediately. This rapidly releases sugar directly into the bloodstream, signaling the pancreas to produce insulin, a hormone that takes the excess sugar out of your bloodstream. Insulin is also a fat-promoting hormone, as you will see. The rapid rise in the blood sugar level causes the pancreas to overreact—so much insulin is produced that the blood sugar level drops precipitously. The result is a quick burst of energy followed by an equally fast fall in energy level.

I bet all of you carbo fans were never told that both simple and complex carbohydrates can be converted into body fat, undermining whatever diet and exercise plan you undertake, if you overeat them. You see, when all kinds of carbohydrates are eaten, even cold cereals or pasta or brown rice, they are converted into glucose (blood sugar), which is used for energy. From here it can go to two places: the muscles or the fat cells. What is not used right away (to fuel exercise) is stored in the liver and muscles as glycogen. When the glycogen storage space is filled, the excess glucose is converted and stored as body fat. How quickly the storage is filled differs with each individual, but we do know one thing. The more physically active you are, the more you will burn the stored carbohydrate source (glycogen) so that there will be room for more.

The more carbohydrates you eat, no matter what the source, the more insulin is released. Insulin is good at moving that glucose off into fat storage, but that creates a sense of shortage in the blood, which sends out the message to increase the blood sugar by, yes, eating more carbohydrates. Fatigue follows every time the blood sugar level drops. So the vicious cycle begins. You suddenly find yourself pigging out on carbohydrates, regardless of whether they're simple or complex, because your blood sugar is constantly low.

But there's another problem with eating too many "fat free" carbohydrates that you've probably never heard about before.

High levels of insulin induced by excessively high carbohydrate diets prevent another pancreatic hormone called glucagon from entering the bloodstream. Glucagon's main job is to unlock the cells of stored body fat so you can utilize them for energy. If there is too much insulin in the bloodstream, your glucagon is held up and you have no way of using up all the fat your body has been storing. This is why you keep craving more and more carbohydrates; you need them for energy because you have no access to the energy you've already got locked in your body in the form of fat.

Overconsumption of carbohydrates can create excess insulin production. Excess insulin production causes sugars to be converted into body fat. In addition, the insulin blocks the fat-burning glucagon from doing its job. The result? More body fat. Every plate of pasta, every breakfast muffin, every box of fat-free cookies, acts like an army, holding back the body fat you already have stored. Instead of using this key resource for energy, you just keep going back to the breadbox. (By the way, although we know about coffee's properties as a stimulant, most of us are not aware of the relationship of caffeine to insulin. Caffeine also indirectly stimulates the production of insulin, thwarting coffee's common use as a tool for weight loss.)

These two hormones, insulin and glucagon, play a vital role in weight loss and weight gain. In fact, it is now recognized that over 75 percent of overweight persons may suffer from a carbohydrate sensitivity. And the problem is getting worse: the less fat food manufacturers put into the foods we eat, the more sugars and simple and processed carbohydrates go into them. Contrary to the idea that you can eat more and weigh less, the more you eat foods that stimulate insulin and suppress glucagon—the more you eat carbohydrates—the more body fat your body is going to store.

Different Sugars and Where They Are Found

Simple sugars, which wreak havoc with our blood sugar levels and fat control systems, are found in many of the foods we commonly eat. Pay attention to the different sugars and where they are found:

- Glucose (dextrose): the main blood sugar in our bodies, our number one energy source; present in many fruits and in the starches of vegetables such as corn.
- Fructose: fruit sugar from fruits, juices, and honey; commercial varieties now use corn as a base. It is twice as sweet as sucrose when added commercially to cold products and about the same sweetness as sucrose in baked goods.
- Sucrose: made up of equal portions of glucose and fructose, this is the most abundant sugar in plants; refined, usually from sugar cane or beets, it has no nutrients. It is best known as table sugar.
- Maltose: malt sugar, formed by the breakdown of starch.
- Lactose: milk sugar; less sweet than sucrose.
- Raw sugar: partially refined sucrose (dirt and plant debris remain, along with some trace minerals).
- Brown sugar: table sugar with molasses coating.
- Powdered sugar: table sugar ground into fine crystals with a small amount of starch added to avoid caking.
- Molasses: residue after crystals of sugar are removed from beet juice or sugar cane; contains a variety of sugars. Blackstrap molasses contains measurable amounts of trace minerals, including calcium and iron.
- Maple sugar: sucrose made from boiling maple sap.
- Honey: natural syrup made up of fructose, glucose, maltose, and sucrose; sweeter than sucrose, it can raise blood sugar levels higher than sucrose does. Its composition, quality, and taste vary, with clover honey generally having more iron than other varieties.

- Corn syrup: derived from corn starch; made up of glucose and maltose.
- High fructose corn syrup: also made from corn starch, with the fructose content increased by enzymes; sweeter than sucrose. It is now used in almost all regular soft drinks.
- Sorbitol, mannitol, and xylitol: synthetic products, sugar alcohols; all are more slowly absorbed than glucose and cause lower insulin responses than either glucose or sucrose. All three have laxative effects on sensitive individuals, however, and cannot be used in great quantity. When sorbitol is used to replace sugars in food products, the end result may contain even more calories because of added fat needed to make the sorbitol more soluble.

How Carbohydrates Can Cause Disease

A high-carbohydrate diet may also be wrong for certain individuals who are prone to diabetes or have a carbohydrate addiction, a term coined by nutritional specialists Drs. Richard and Rachel Heller of the Mt. Sinai School of Medicine in New York. According to the Hellers, about 75 percent of all overweight individuals have carbohydrate addiction or insulin resistance, a condition created by an imbalance in the amount of insulin, which controls the body's blood sugar.

Normal individuals produce just the right amount of insulin when carbohydrates are consumed, for reasons still not completely understood by scientists. A person who has carbohydrate addiction or insulin resistance produces more insulin than is necessary. How do you know if you have an insulin problem? In addition to a constant craving for carbohydrate-rich foods and a difficulty dropping extra pounds, you experience excessive thirst, excessive need to urinate, mood swings, fatigue in late morning or midafternoon, and light-headedness. If these sound familiar, they are also the symptoms of diabetes, also known as hyperinsulinemia. (The concept of insulin resistance was introduced over 20 years ago by Dr. Robert Atkins, who called insulin excess "the hidden force behind many major illnesses, from diabetes to heart disease.") Excessive insulin levels in the blood then create even more hunger and cravings for high-carbo foods (like bread, snack foods and sweets) and result in fat storage, not to mention an inability to burn the fat you already have.

The best indicators for insulin resistance are triglyceride levels above 200 and HDL cholesterol below 35.

What about Sugar Substitutes?

When we talk about carbohydrates, of course, we're talking about sugar. Since we know that sugar will elevate insulin levels, creating the risk of obesity, diabetes, and heart disease, what about artificial sweeteners? I remember well the story of Jan Smith, from *Idea Today* (September, 1991), who at 35 taught bench and low-impact aerobics and circuit training. She also drank a lot of diet soda sweetened with NutraSweet and ate a lot of sugar-free foods, also containing NutraSweet. Although she seemed to be fine, Jan suddenly began gaining weight, topping out at 30 pounds above her usual weight. She began losing her hair, her skin broke out, and she suffered from headaches, heart palpitations, and mood swings severe enough to be suicidal. Her cholesterol sharply increased and she developed ear and vision problems, shooting pains in her limbs, and problems with her menstrual cycle.

Jan worked out even harder to try to combat the weight gain, but then her blood pressure shot up. Doctors finally diagnosed Graves' disease and told her she had to have her thyroid removed or she would die. Fortunately, Jan had a background in environmental science. She began to investigate, and discovered her body lacked chromium, an essential mineral that aspartame (also known as Equal and NutraSweet) removes from the body. She linked her symptoms, including—surprisingly—her sudden weight *gain,* to the use of diet foods laced with NutraSweet that she had begun using in earnest about 18 months earlier. Within a month of quitting the NutraSweet and all the products it was found in, Jan's symptoms (and the extra weight) disappeared.

Many people, in an attempt to avoid sugar, use sugar substitutes. Aspartame (known as NutraSweet and Equal) is an ingredient in more than 3,000 foods, including diet sodas and diet foods like sugar-free yogurt and powdered drink mixes. Toothpaste, sugar-free gum, pudding, packaged desserts, dietetic foods, sweets for diabetics, and just about any product you can think of that used to have sugar in it now may have aspartame instead. Aspartame is a combination of three substances: the amino acid phenylalanine, aspartic acid, and methanol (wood alcohol). Each of these has been known to cause serious side effects. Phenylalanine, for example, lowers or blocks production of serotonin, an amine that sends messages from the pineal gland in the brain. This blockage is a potential cause of carbohydrate cravings, PMS symptoms, insomnia, and mood swings.

In some circumstances, people may be getting excessively high levels of methanol; it is estimated that on a hot day after exercising, if you drink three 12-ounce cans of diet soda, you could easily be consuming as much as eight times the Environmental Protection Agency's recommended limits for methanol consumption. Exercise can be a component in the dangers of aspartame. Jan, who now avidly supports the Aspartame Consumer Safety Network (ACSN) in Dallas, Texas (214) 352-4268, pointed out that aspartame and its by-products (including free-form wood alcohol) can race through the system of a very fit person who has a high metabolic rate. When you work out, the activity of all your body systems is intensified, and so are reactions to whatever is in the body at the time. Ironically, it seems that fitness instructors are particularly prone to drinking diet soda with NutraSweet in between classes, and so may be in the most danger.

Far from being the answer to the sugar problem, aspartame has instead spurred numerous complaints from unsuspecting consumers, which now represent 80 to 85 percent of all food complaints registered with the Food and Drug Administration. Among 73 different symptoms are attributed to aspartame use, including dizziness, headaches, loss of equilibrium, ear problems, hemorrhaging of the eyes, and visual impairment. The dangers of artificial sweeteners have become so widespread that the Aspartame Consumer Safety Network now offers scientific information and acts as a clearinghouse of information on adverse reactions. Three Senate hearings have been conducted on the safety of aspartame, and the Center for Science in the Public Interest (CSPI) in Washington, D.C., now lists it as the third-worst additive. Since you never know how much you could be ingesting, I suggest you completely avoid any foods with added NutraSweet or any other artificial sweetener.

The Problems of Too Much Fruit

While you may now be more conscious of the way in which simple sugars and excessive carbos promote body fat, you may not realize that certain fruits and fruit juices can also promote body fat. Yes, even those health food "natural" cookies and other desserts that are sweetened with fruit juice concentrates instead of sugar can be as fattening as those made with white sugar, if they are eaten in excess.

You see, fructose, the major ingredient in fruits and fruit juices, is a simple sugar. It does have some benefits for certain individuals. Unlike other sugars, it is initially absorbed more slowly into the bloodstream, and so creates a more level blood glucose than other simple sugars. The absorption of other sugars (white sugar and honey, for example) causes a fast rise in blood sugar, with the familiar sugar rush and the resulting crash, followed by hunger. Fructose provides a steady stream of energy instead of a rush, which is why it has been recommended by some for diabetics. But fructose is also known for *stimulating fat storage!*

Fructose goes directly to the liver, the only organ that can metabolize it, where it is converted into triglycerides, a fat. High triglyceride levels, especially in women, are associated with heart disease. I have counseled many women who eat a lot of fruit, fruit juices, and fruit-juice-sweetened snacks, believing these are good substitutes for refined sugars. In fact, the results have been disastrous. Many of these women were unable to lose weight until I limited them to one to two pieces of fresh fruit a day and eliminated all fruit juices and fruit-juice-sweetened snacks from their diets.

When eaten in a concentrated source, even by drinking just one glass of fruit juice, the conversion process of fruit into glucose and then into fat can be magnified. Many people have been misled about fructose; they believe they can eat large quantities of fruit with few of sugar's side effects. Because of its high concentration of the simple sugar fructose, fruit juice (even the naturally extracted, unsweetened, organic, freshly squeezed variety) eventually *causes the same reaction* that other simple carbohydrates do: the peak and valley syndrome of blood sugar level. Another side effect of a diet high in fructose is that it can elevate the uric acid level in the blood, which leads to gout, a condition often erroneously blamed on excess protein.

All of these negative fruit effects are magnified in the form of high-fructose corn syrup—common in processed foods and soft drinks. In fact, a USDA 1993 study found that fructose increases artery-clogging LDL cholesterol.

Now, you know of some problems associated with overconsumption of sugar, such as cavities and mood swings. What you may not be aware of is that *any* sugar, whether it is table sugar, honey, glucose, fructose, or even that in freshly squeezed orange juice, has a negative effect on the ability of the body to fight disease. The immune system is so sensitive to sugars of any kind that its effectiveness is immediately reduced by half when sugars are consumed, even in as small an amount as one glass of juice. (All forms of alcohol—beer, wine, liquor, and liqueurs—have such a high sugar content and such a minimal amount of nutrients that they, too, act as simple sugars in the body, hastening the fat-storage process, depressing your immune system, wildly unbalancing your blood sugar, and filling you up with empty calories to boot.)

The Relationship between Carbohydrates and Exercise

Certainly we all know how important exercise is to help us lose weight. One of its forgotten benefits, however, is that it can also cut back insulin levels in the blood. As I have already stated, it's only when insulin levels decrease (and glucagon production increases) that you can tap into your stored body fat. To lose weight, and access stored body fat, you need a slow and steady release of energy, which you have when the carbohydrates in your diet are balanced with protein and certain healthy fats, as you will see later. If your diet is high in simple carbohydrates, insulin is increased and some of the carbohydrate itself is used for energy, while its excess gets deposited in the tissue as more fat. Interestingly enough, this information has finally made it into studies on athletes, who in the past have preferred high-carbohydrate diets for fast energy. An eight-week research study in California in 1993 concluded that athletes may actually perform better on a diet lower in carbohydrates and higher in protein.

Runners tested in the study (nine men and nine women) received a higher proportion of their energy from stored body fat when their diet was adjusted to contain more protein. As I've just explained, this stored body fat is unavailable when we eat a lot of carbohydrates but is easily accessible when we follow a diet with more protein in it. Protein also provides better appetite control than carbohydrates because it enters the blood system more slowly than carbohydrates. Another benefit of reducing carbohydrate intake that was found in the study is that the good HDL cholesterol increases when insulin levels go down; carbohydrates cause insulin levels to go up, thus possibly lowering the good HDL cholesterol and raising the bad LDL cholesterol.

Complex and Processed Carbohydrates— Two Different Things

When you eat **complex carbohydrates** (such as vegetables and legumes), the whole process is slowed down considerably. In fact, because of their complex molecular structure, these foods are far less likely to turn into body fat, *with one very important exception.* Complex carbohydrate foods made from *grains* (even those made from whole-grain flour) like breads, pasta, and bagels as well as rice cakes and puffed cold cereals—the most popular complex carbohydrates—react more like *simple* sugars in the body because of the processing the original grain has gone through.

This means that eating whole-grain flour products like bread or pasta instead of the whole grains themselves (like steamed barley, buckwheat, quinoa, amaranth, millet, old fashioned rolled oats, etc.) is going to cause the same situation in the body that simple sugars do. Absorbed quickly into the bloodstream as glucose, these processed-grain products stimulate the pancreas into overproducing that fat-promoting hormone, insulin, which starts the fat storage process. Again, glucagon production, which would open up fat cells you already have as an energy source, is suppressed. In fact, we might almost consider processed-grain foods to be in their own category of carbohydrate: the **processed carbohydrate.**

With the refining process, nutritious whole grains once high in vitamins, minerals, and fiber are converted into processed foods that have a long shelf life but act like simple carbohydrates in the body. Far from helping you lose weight, *they easily break down into sugars stored as body fat.* In addition, a diet high in processed carbohydrates like bread and pasta (or simple carbohydrates like fruit and sugary desserts) results in increased hunger and food cravings, raises triglyceride levels, and lowers the levels of all amino acids except tryptophan, which causes drowsiness.

The important thing to remember about this process is that the more simple and processed carbohydrates you eat, the more insulin you secrete. The more insulin you secrete, the less your own body fat is used for energy and the more carbohydrate excess gets turned to fat. Except perhaps in the case of power athletes who spend several hours every day in hard physical training, most of us are not using up all the energy that the high-carbohydrate diet supplies; all that excess carbo energy just gets turned to fat, regardless of whether we are insulin resistant or not, because many of us are simply eating too much of a good thing.

Even though many healthy diet plans call for an increase in complex carbohydrates, they rarely distinguish between vegetables and processed carbos like grain products. Reducing or eliminating the use of processed carbohydrates and increasing the amount of complex carbohydrates you eat in the form of *vegetables* and some *whole grains* (one to two servings a day), regardless of your metabolic type, blood type, and ancestry, is one of the biggest steps you can take to effectively lose weight and stay healthy.

The Glycemic Effects of Foods on Health

Research that has absolutely gone ignored in conventional nutritional wisdom is the study of the "glycemic index," which shows the difference between foods that offer a consistent level of endurance and those that cause a fast burnout. The glycemic index is the rate at which a carbohydrate breaks down to be released as glucose into the bloodstream. Remember, release too fast, and you get the fast high/fast crash blood sugar syndrome, as well as the attendant problems of insulin secretion and glucagon suppression. Releasing glucose at a slower rate can provide the brain and the body with a steady stream of energy over several hours, a rate preferable for most of us to maintain energy throughout the day. This also prevents fatigue. The only time we might want that burst of energy might be just before or immediately after an intense workout; otherwise, we're better off with that slow, steady stream.

Foods with a high glycemic index are foods that release glucose into the bloodstream quickly. Here are some examples of high-glycemic foods: rice cakes (133), white bread (100), Grape-Nuts (98), honey (87), white potatoes (81), All-Bran cereal (74). These foods cause glucose to enter the bloodstream quickly, resulting in the fast high/fast crash syndrome as well as the overproduction of insulin and eventual fat storage. Foods with a low glycemic index, offering a steady stream of energy, include yams (51), grapes (45), whole-grain rye bread (42), apples (39), lentils (29), cherries (23), and soybeans (15). (You'll find a complete list in the chapter on exercise, Chapter 7.)

What startled me about the glycemic index rating of a food is that it has nothing to do with whether it is a simple or complex carbohydrate. It has more to do with the ease with which a food is digested, the quantity of fiber, and the form in which the food is eaten. Cooking makes a starch more digestible, which therefore raises its glycemic index higher than if it were raw.

During my nutritional education, I was taught that the complex carbohydrates, because they are more complex in biochemical structure, release more slowly into the system. In fact, the glycemic index suggests that's not the case. Even certain complex carbohydrates, such as white potatoes, carrots, and oat bran, which all have a high glycemic index rating, release energy into the bloodstream very quickly. If you're going to be doing a lot of exercise, they provide fast energy, but if you don't use it, you'll get a blood sugar peak and then a valley.

One way to slow down this quick glucose release is to eat a high glycemic-index carbohydrate (like brown rice, for example) with a more slowly digested food (like chicken), which has a leveling action on the glucose release. Don't forget that the protein in chicken spurs the production of glucagon, which helps you mobilize your stored body fat.

Problems with Grains

Besides the creation or storage of body fat and the other factors I've mentioned, there are other side effects from a diet too high in certain carbohydrates. Remember, grain products are fairly new foods to the human diet. Dr. Richard Kunin, an ortho-molecular physician from San Francisco, says it best: "Grains are really Johnny-come-latelies on the nutritional scene. Meats, fruits, beans, seeds, nuts and vegetables have had a considerably longer historical alliance with the human gut. Almost as if to make up for lost time, grain has deluged man's diet and this excess increasingly appears to have something to do with common major and minor ailments."

Grains and grain products are associated with a whole range of problems, including carbohydrate addiction and yeast infections, or candidiasis. Sensitivity to grains that contain gluten (the protein fraction of the grain, which gives it its resilient quality), mainly wheat and rye, and to a lesser extent, oats and barley, is known as gluten intolerance or celiac/sprue disease. Gluten intolerance can be the hidden cause of diarrhea, poor appetite, anemia, foul-smelling stools, cramps, and muscle spasms. Another side effect of gluten intolerance is malabsorption of vitamins, resulting in chronic deficiencies that can be the cause of depression, fatigue, and lack of motivation as well as more serious diseases like cancer. Other problems that can be due to gluten intolerance include disorders of the adrenal, parathyroid, and pituitary glands, vague aches and pains, intestinal gas and bloating, arthritis and connective tissue disorders, alcoholism, breast cancer, and gallbladder problems. Gluten intolerance has even been implicated in multiple sclerosis, rheumatoid arthritis, and schizophrenia.

I have counseled many professional, sophisticated women who keep up with all the latest dietary and nutrition information. Most of them have subscribed to the low-fat, high-carbohydrate advice, following the suggestions to a T. Unfortunately, they very quickly start to experience symptoms they can't explain. They feel bloated several hours after eating. They have severe PMS, with cramps and heavy bleeding. They have irregular bowel movements. They find they bruise easily, and have lots of bone pains. They go through months of suffering because they refuse to pay attention to the signals their bodies are giving them, that they just are not doing well with all these grains. They were so concerned with nutrition that they wanted to follow the perfect diet 100 percent but they lost touch with what their bodies were telling them. Most times, your body does not lie.

Candidiasis, or *Candida albicans* overgrowth, is another form of fallout from a diet heavy in carbohydrates, including whole-grain products made with yeast as well as sweets, fruit, and alcohol. Normally not a problem in healthy individuals, the natural yeast *Candida* can overgrow in the intestines when the immune system is depressed. This yeast growth is usually controlled by beneficial intestinal bacteria, but those organisms are killed off when antibiotics are taken or are eaten secondhand through antibiotic-treated meat. Without that friendly flora, the yeast multiplies, causing chronic vaginal yeast infections as well as a host of symptoms throughout the body: fatigue, sinus infections, headaches, gastrointestinal discomfort and bloating, earaches and infections, and others.

I have counseled more women suffering from chronic yeast infections than practically any other problem. Most of them are eating a high-carbohydrate diet, at the expense of protein and essential oils, in order to reduce dietary fat. They load up on yeast-promoting spices and condiments like mustard, vinegar, and soy sauce to compensate for the lack of flavor fat provides. They also eat excessive amounts of crackers, pastas, muffins, and breads, as well as natural fruits and fruit juices to satisfy their increasing sugar cravings. They've cut out red meat, eggs, and healthy fats from their diet. The result is an overgrowth of yeast in the system and difficulty in losing weight. Many researchers are now suggesting a connection between an overgrowth of yeast and chronic fatigue syndrome, as well as infection with the intestinal parasite *Giardia lamblia* (giardiasis). (See Chapter 8, Living in the Nineties, for a deeper discussion of both candidiasis and parasites and treatment information.)

You must now be asking, if grain-based carbohydrates, which are presented as the foundation of today's current nutritional standard, are such a problem for the human body, why are they being so heavily touted? To answer this question, we need to consider some important health trends of the past two decades.

Starting with the 1971 publication of Frances Moore Lappé's *Diet for a Small Planet,* which advocated combining beans and grains to replace animal protein in the diet, grains have been elevated to supernutrition status, as well as being considered a spiritually conscious food choice. The rise in vegetarianism and the many cookbooks prominently featuring grains that followed also contributed to the growth in carbohydrate consumption. Nathan Pritikin transformed the image of carbohydrates from a lowly staple to a sure way to coronary health. Pasta underwent a similar transformation, from peasant fare to glamorous status, highly approved by dietitians for weight control and as an energy source for athletes. In addition, recommendations to decrease fats and cholesterol in the diet have led many people to add more and more grains to the diet as a substitute for other foods.

Grains have a legitimate place in the balanced diet. After all, they are a good source of fiber and the B vitamins. The problem is that we have been overemphasizing grains. The idea that a diet heavy in grains is good for everybody is a myth. This is the foundation of the theme of this book, that one universal food plan does not work for everybody.

Generally speaking, carbohydrates are a prime source of energy, as well as fiber, vitamins, and minerals. However, variety, moderation, and balance are the key nutritional watchwords. When you vary the foods you eat, you automatically reduce the foods you have been overloading on, like carbohydrates. Most people will do well to *cut back on the simple carbohydrates* (especially fruit and sugary foods combined with fat) *as well as the processed carbohydrates* (like breads, pastas, and other flour-based dishes). This way, you can control your fat-promoting insulin production, assist your fat-burning glucagon production, and achieve a balanced blood sugar.

Stick mainly to *complex carbohydrates* from legumes and vegetables, such as lentils, chick peas, corn, and squash, which can help you reduce grain overload. Learn to snack on nuts and seeds instead of breads, muffins, and crackers.

If you think you might be gluten intolerant, you can substitute rice, millet, and buckwheat for gluten-containing wheat, rye, oats, and barley. Another great grain to try is spelt, an ancient grain related to wheat that is much lower in gluten. Spelt is a tough grain that requires fewer pesticides to grow because its tough outer shell protects it from insects and disease. It's higher in fiber and protein than wheat, and helps improve digestion and normalize cholesterol.

Food for Thought

Do you feel like you could eat a whole loaf of bread? Do you love big, steaming plates of pasta morning, noon, and night?

Do you feel tired or hungry in the midafternoon? Does your stomach feel bloated several hours after eating?

Do you find yourself eating every two hours if you've started your day with a sweet roll or Danish?

If so, you may be carbohydrate-sensitive and a perfect candidate for a carbohydrate-reduced diet.

3

Protein: The Body's Foundation

Another important building block of the human body is protein. It has gotten an ill-deserved reputation over the last several years, primarily because meats laden with saturated fats have been associated with heart disease. Since at least the beginning of this century, the American diet has traditionally been heavy on protein, particularly meat, eggs, and dairy products. It has only been in the latter part of the twentieth century that these protein staples have been considered a culprit in the rise of coronary health problems. As you'll see later in this chapter, I believe this negative assessment of protein is not completely true, but due to its widespread notoriety, I now find myself reviewing food records of diet-conscious clients who are alarmingly deficient in protein.

I remember all too well the case of Virginia, who often bragged about her no-fat diet. Her food diary revealed that she had eliminated all animal protein, dairy foods, and eggs from her life. She snacked on vegetable-based mini-meals all day long and light frozen entrees were her usual meals. At nine o'clock at night, she would go into munchie mayhem, filling up on frozen yogurt, yogurt-covered candy, and fat-free cookies sweetened with fruit juice. Virginia was also very moody, with a short temper, but it wasn't until she started seeing clumps of hair on her pillow that she knew something had to change. Her lack of dietary protein had completely undermined her attempts at perfect health.

Fatigue, mental confusion, irritability, loss of hair, thinning skin, brittle nails, lack of sex drive, and constant food cravings are the common complaints of people with protein deficiency like Virginia. They are trying to satisfy their body's resulting hunger for protein with sugary foods and fruit. In fact, sugar consumption skyrockets in this increasingly common scenario. Even with increased awareness of the dangers of dietary fat, sugar intake in this country has quietly crept up to 152 pounds per person per year, up 10 pounds from a decade ago.

All the Roles Protein Plays

Protein plays an important role in the body. It is essential for tissue growth and repair and for forming neurotransmitters in the brain. It boosts the metabolic rate, enhances the immune system with the production of antibodies, and provides all the necessary animo acids to the body. It dictates the catabolic/anabolic cycle of the body, in which muscle tissue is broken down (catabolism) during strenuous physical activity and then rebuilt (anabolism). When protein is increased in the diet, the body forms new muscle.

One of protein's most specific functions is to stimulate the production of the hormone *glucagon*. Glucagon's job, if you recall from the chapter on carbohydrates, is to open up the cells of stored fat already in the body for use as a fuel source. What this means is that eating protein in the form of poultry, fish, and red meat actually helps us lose weight by allowing our bodies to burn off its stored fat.

Protein builds new cells to replace those that are constantly lost in day-to-day living, such as hair and skin cells. Protein also raises the metabolic rate. If you have a slow metabolism, or feel sluggish, increasing protein in your diet will help speed it up. You'll have more energy and better endurance. The higher your metabolic rate, the faster you are able to burn off fat stores and the better you utilize the energy foods you eat.

Another function of protein has to do with fluid balance. Proteins in the blood attract water molecules, regulating the amount of water in between cells, within cells, and inside the capillaries, veins, and arteries. When there is not enough protein in the diet, the blood becomes deficient in protein; water then can leak out from the cell walls to the spaces in between cells where it can't be extracted by the kidneys. The result of a *low-protein diet* (especially one that is too high in carbohydrates) is *bloating, water retention,* and *water weight gain.*

Proteins also strengthen the immune system by producing antibodies that combat disease. Antibodies deactivate intruders such as viruses and bacteria. If protein intake is low, then your antibody protection is low. Proteins also assist in the function of lymphocytes and leukocytes, which promote immunity at the cellular level. When the number of leukocytes decreases, cellular metabolism is slowed and resistance to bacterial invasion is weakened.

With all the good things protein does for the body, why would anyone not want to eat it? Many are avoiding protein today because they've been given the wrong information about fat and have connected that wrong information to protein.

Misinformation about Protein and Fat

What, then, is the relationship between protein (in the form of meat) and heart disease? After all, haven't diet gurus and heart surgeons been promoting a general cutback in our intake of red meat to protect the population from heart disease? Unfortunately, beef has been taking the rap for another dietary culprit, the artificial and processed trans fats found in margarine and hydrogenated oils. I'll discuss the dangers of trans fats in the next chapter. Protein, in and of itself, is not a direct component of heart disease. The problem with today's protein-rich red meat is due to the way in which cattle are currently raised and has nothing to do with the protein beef contains.

Years ago, most beef was range-fed on large grasslands. A fatty acid called oleic acid naturally accumulated in the muscles of the cattle. Now, most beef cattle are fed grains and fattened up in feed lots with the help of the growth hormone stilbestrol. As a result, their muscles store up a different kind of fat, called stearic acid. Stearic acid promotes production of the bad LDL cholesterol, the one we're always recommended to lower.

Now is as good a time as any to tackle the cholesterol issue, although I will go into it in greater detail in the next chapter. Much has been said about high cholesterol levels, which are supposedly caused by high-cholesterol diets. In reality, many studies have not been able to prove any relation at all between cholesterol in the diet and serum cholesterol levels. One study done on 4,000 people in Tecumseh, Michigan, in 1976 determined only that there was a correlation between weight and cholesterol levels. The people who were overweight had high cholesterol levels, but their cholesterol levels were not affected by eating a high-cholesterol diet.

The Framingham Heart Study, a famous ongoing study that has lasted more than 60 years, is designed to investigate the risk factors in heart disease. Although researchers did find that serum cholesterol (cholesterol in the blood) correlated strongly with heart disease, they were unable to prove any correlation between cholesterol in the diet and heart disease. Specifically, they found no relationship between the consumption of high-cholesterol foods like eggs, fats, or meat and heart disease. Blood serum cholesterol does appear to have a relationship to heart disease, but not to cholesterol in the diet. And high serum cholesterol can be created by a diet lacking essential fats and a diet high in sugar and carbohydrates. Heart disease is also correlated to hypertension, cigarette smoking, diabetes, the ratio between good HDL and bad LDL cholesterol, excess weight, and lack of exercise.)

Keep in mind that some cholesterol is necessary in the diet: if we don't eat enough of it, our bodies actually accelerate cholesterol production. Cholesterol has some very vital functions in our bodies. That is why our cells manufacture it if it drops to a low level in our system. Cholesterol is involved in the synthesis of sex hormones, the myelin sheath (the coating around nerves), vitamin D, and bile (involved in the digestion of fats). No matter what you eat, your cholesterol levels can actually increase under stress because in times of stress, the body actually produces more cholesterol for the adrenal glands (our stress busters) to fight with. It's no wonder that cholesterol levels of accountants seem to go up around April 15!

Dairy: Not the Answer to Every Body's Protein and Calcium Needs

The two main sources of the most biologically complete dietary protein are meat and eggs, which have been misrepresented as harmful by the media the past several years. *Avoiding any source of protein is not the way to reduce body fat, cholesterol levels, or the risk of heart disease.* Conversely, increasing dairy products in the diet in order to increase calcium intake may not be the boon many of us think it is. Remember my previous discussion about the new foods in our diet? Just like grains, dairy products are a recent addition to the human diet that came along with domesticated animals about 10,000 years ago. Several million years before that, mother's milk was the only dairy product humans ate, and they only consumed that during the first year or two of life.

Dairy products, especially low-fat cheeses and yogurt, are foods touted as high in protein, vitamins, and minerals that could replace meat in the average diet. The calcium and vitamin D content of dairy products makes them particularly popular; women at risk for osteoporosis in their later years are urged to incorporate dairy products into their diets on a regular basis.

For the majority of the world's adult population, though, milk is a source of calcium they cannot biochemically utilize. At some point between the ages of 18 months and 4 years, most people stop producing the intestinal enzyme called lactase, which is needed to break down milk sugar, or lactose. This normal process is similar to that of the animal world, where the lactase enzyme becomes unnecessary shortly after weaning. The resulting lack of lactase causes undigested lactose from eating dairy products to move into the colon, where it ferments, resulting in bloating, gas, cramps, and, in some cases, diarrhea. Humans are the only animals that continue to drink milk after weaning, yet worldwide, far more people suffer from lactose intolerance than do not, and therefore cannot benefit from the calcium in milk.

Think about your own ancestral heritage, and you may find out why milk and milk products don't always agree with you. A high proportion of African Americans, Greeks, Arabs, Israeli Jews, Ashkenazi Jews, and Orientals are lactose intolerant.

Another aspect of the dairy-based calcium dilemma is that if calcium is not mobilized into the bones with the aid of magnesium, it may collect in soft tissues and cause calcium deposits and arthritis. Although popular attention has been on calcium for several years, an equally important mineral is magnesium, which optimally should be taken in equal proportion to calcium. A magnesium deficiency will prevent the chemical action of calcium absorption, and it is the transfer of calcium from our blood into our bones via magnesium that helps prevent osteoarthritis and osteoporosis.

Dairy products contain nine times as much calcium as magnesium. Our evolving human ancestors had a ready supply of magnesium in the form of nuts, seeds, beans, and vegetables and therefore did not develop a storage mechanism for this mineral. But because they did not have high-calcium foods like dairy products readily available, their bodies did evolve to store calcium effectively. Because of this storage mechanism, a little bit of calcium goes a long way in the body. As I have mentioned before, our bodies are not biochemically different from our Stone Age ancestors of 40,000 years ago. We still store calcium more efficiently than magnesium, so we don't have to eat nearly as much as the dairy industry has conditioned us to believe. We don't have to drink several glasses of milk every day and we don't have to eat a lot of cheese. Calcium has even been added to unlikely substances, such as orange juice. Some antacids (like Tums) are now being promoted as sources of calcium.

However, magnesium hasn't received the hype calcium has and, consequently, we don't eat *enough* magnesium-rich foods, which would help the mobilization of calcium into the bones. Magnesium can be found in many foods such as leafy green vegetables, nuts, seeds, and sea vegetables. Symptoms of a lack of magnesium in the diet include nervousness, insomnia, depression, brittle bones, and becoming startled at the smallest noise. We also deplete what magnesium we do consume by a diet high in sugar and alcohol, which increases magnesium excretion through the urine. Even if you eat yogurt every day for its calcium content, you may not be absorbing the calcium well if you don't also eat foods with magnesium. If you've been avoiding almonds because you think they're too high in fat, think again; almonds are very high in magnesium, and therefore would be very helpful as an adjunct to your yogurt. Oriental and Indian diets contain little or no dairy products and, therefore, may provide a more balanced calcium/magnesium ratio. It is worthwhile to note that neither osteoporosis nor arthritis is a major health problem in these cultures, possibly because of this more ideal calcium/magnesium balance.

Eggs—the Good Guys

Eggs have been called a bad guy because of their high cholesterol content, but I say eggs are the good guys. As a source of complete protein as well as vitamins, minerals, and amino acids, eggs can't be topped. Eggs are one of the only dietary sources of the sulfur-bearing amino acid L-cysteine, which is so essential for healthy nails and skin and lustrous hair. The protein of eggs comes closest to matching the protein pattern best used by the body.

Many of us have been avoiding eggs in our diet because of the cholesterol propaganda that has been attached to them in recent years. As I mentioned above, the evidence for the belief that high levels of dietary cholesterol always raise blood cholesterol is underwhelming, at best. Studies from the University of California at Los Angeles, the University of Missouri, and other sources find no correlation between cholesterol in the diet and heart attack rates. In a year-long Canadian study of both the Pritikin low-fat diet and the American Heart Association limited-fat diet, neither diet lowered blood cholesterol levels in patients who had the beginning stages of vascular disease. After following the diets of 912 residents of Framingham, Massachusetts, the Boston University Framingham Heart Study found that there was no association between egg consumption and deaths from coronary heart disease. There were also no significant differences in the actual blood cholesterol levels between people who ate several eggs a week (7 to 24) and those who ate only a few (0 to 2½). So why have eggs gotten a bad reputation?

We've been operating under the simplistic notion that dietary cholesterol equals elevated blood cholesterol, which equals increased risk of heart disease. Now we know better. In fact, the original study that put eggs on the list of dangerous foods was done about 50 years ago. It was sponsored by the Cereal Institute and was conducted using dried egg yolk powder, not the freshly cooked, fried, or poached eggs most of us eat. Recent refutations of that study have pointed out that dried yolk powder in and of itself is toxic to blood vessels because it has been oxidized, which is a metabolic process that renders fats dangerous to the human body. No subsequent studies have been able to prove any cholesterol dangers—or any other kind of dangers—from eating eggs.

The good news is that if you've been avoiding eggs because of their high cholesterol content, you have no reason to avoid them anymore. High cholesterol levels in foods do not turn into high cholesterol in the bloodstream. Eggs happen to be high in lecithin, which is a cholesterol-lowering agent. Biochemically speaking, eggs are a healthy source of protein that is a convenient, natural, and unprocessed food. Eggs will satisfy your hunger so you don't have to fill up on high levels of carbohydrates—a far more deleterious habit than regular egg consumption. Cholesterol content should not be an issue even if you eat one or two eggs or more every day.

Another positive aspect of the egg to take into account is its germinative property. An egg is like a plant seed, containing all the essentials for the growth of an organism. One of the standards of nutrition is that germinative foods are the most nutritious. Therefore, roe, seeds, and sprouts are fine items to include in your diet.

The Vegetarian Diet and Biochemical Individuality

Meanwhile, an additional aspect of the entire discussion of proteins is whether or not animal proteins are *necessary* components of the human diet, or whether they can be adequately substituted with other foods. Spiritual, philosophical, ecological, and economic reasons for abstaining from meat have been added to the promoted health values of the vegetarian diet. However, based on years of personal counseling and my own experience as a vegetarian, as well as strongly supportive scientific research, I don't believe that everybody should be a vegetarian, or even that everybody *can* be a vegetarian. Some people, because of their genetic inheritance and ancestry, are better designed biologically than others for a vegetarian or near-vegetarian diet. However, I believe everyone would be more healthy physically if they ate some meat.

I believe that animal protein plays a significant role in the human diet, even though the amounts necessary for optimal health and weight levels are different for different people. Once again, the key to how much meat we should eat is in our biochemical individuality and should be based on our metabolic rate, our ancestry, our genetic inheritance, and our blood type.

My Experience with a Vegetarian Diet

Documented advantages to the vegetarian or vegan diet (which includes no animal tissue at all, including dairy products) are impressive and persuasive. They include a lower risk of heart disease, reduced blood pressure, decreased cancer risk, lower incidence of osteoporosis, a lower incidence of gallstones, lower percentage of body fat, and a decreased risk of prostate cancer.

For these as well as spiritual and philosophical reasons, some 12.4 million Americans now describe themselves as vegetarians. For these same reasons, I became a vegetarian when I was in college. I followed a natural hygiene-type regimen for almost a year, including abundant juicing and meals of raw foods. I knew that avoiding animal protein was not the only answer to cleansing my body and my soul, so when the concept of matching complementary proteins was introduced, I worked very hard at combining foods and planning balanced meals. A healthy vegetarian diet supposedly made up for the lack of animal protein through a formula of combined foods to create complete proteins out of incomplete proteins. Combinations such as grains with legumes (rice and beans) and grains with nuts and seeds (peanut butter sandwich) were frequent meals for me. I drank a lot of carrot juice and ate a lot of raw vegetables, brown rice, seeds, and nuts. I ate no dairy, no eggs, and no beef, chicken, or fish.

I started this program while spending a summer in Israel, interning with a natural hygiene doctor. By about the middle of my senior year, my hair started falling out and I couldn't stand the noise in my dorm. My nerves were on edge, I lost about 20 pounds, and my skin broke out. My parents were very upset at my deteriorating physical condition, but no one could convince me to eat animal products. I felt like I knew all the answers, I could recite them in my sleep: the length of the human intestines, the size of the teeth, and all the significant longevity and health research had convinced me not only of the necessity but of the moral correctness of a vegetarian diet.

After all, a meat-eating animal (like a tiger, lion, or bear) has relatively short intestines that are about three times the length of its trunk—which is perfect for quick elimination of flesh food. A human, on the other hand, has intestines that are about 12 times its trunk length and are designed for more involved digestion, assimilation, and elimination. A meat-eating animal has teeth that are pointed, long, and sharp, while the majority of human teeth (the molars) are shaped specifically for grinding foods like cereals, seed, grains, and legumes. The human also has some incisors (that are good for vegetable cutting) and the smallest number of canines, those sharp, long, pointed teeth that carnivores have.

Despite all of these reasons, being a vegetarian back in the early 1970s—unlike being one today—was neither socially acceptable nor politically correct. I never went out to eat with my friends and, in fact, I was in danger of losing them because I was so intent on converting them to vegetarianism. I was still popular in the dorm, however, because I had a little refrigerator in my room, which became the storehouse for the dorm's snacks. Much to my own embarrassment then and even now, I used to wake up in the middle of the night so ravenously hungry from my severe diet that I would stuff myself with tahini (sesame seed paste) and honey.

This gives me the opportunity to give a true confession. I've waited all these years to tell one of my close friends—Linda Hershkowitz—that, in fact, it was *I* who ate her stash of organic tomatoes that were mysteriously missing from the refrigerator time and time again when she came to get them!

It was not until I saw a photograph of myself and realized how unhealthy I looked (as well as the experience of a nighttime foray into a dormmate's room to binge on a stash of raw honey) that I knew I needed help. In retrospect, I feel now that I lost the joy of my senior year, a time that should have been a lot of fun for me. I called my parents in the middle of the night and told them that I had to see a doctor right away. With the help of a friend, we located a physician who specialized in nutrition. He put me on megavitamins and insisted I begin eating chicken. That was the first step on my road back to health.

Possible Problems of a Vegetarian Diet

Unfortunately, today I see my own experience being mirrored by hundreds of my own clients. Their high-carbohydrate, low-fat, low- to no-animal-protein diets have led to a host of debilitating symptoms that I've mentioned earlier, particularly menstrual irregularities among the women. I remember one client in particular who could be a stand-in for all my clients struggling with a vegetarian or near-vegetarian diet. She contacted me only after she realized she had stopped menstruating. Our nutrition review revealed that she was a very busy woman, constantly on the run, who felt she was being virtuous in her diet by eliminating red meat. She was careful to eat a lot of grains and beans as well as soy products for their reported high-protein content. Unfortunately, as a blood type O with a very fast metabolism, her body was not biologically suited for such a spartan diet. It was only after I convinced her to start eating fish as an experiment that she started maintaining a regular menstrual cycle once again.

Although this wasn't the case with this particular client, one of the biggest problems among people who choose a vegetarian diet is a lack of attention paid to the time-consuming but necessary effort of creating a well-balanced, nutritious diet without meat and animal proteins. If great care isn't taken to make sure they get optimal amounts of certain vitamins and minerals, vegetarians can develop numerous nutrient deficiencies that can lead to ill health.

Zinc Insufficiency in Vegetarians

One of the most common deficiencies I see in vegetarians is a lack of zinc, a crucial mineral for proper immune, reproductive, and blood sugar functioning. Zinc is found in the highest amounts in red meats, poultry, and shellfish, so vegans miss out on the best sources of this important mineral. In addition, traditional vegetarian meals consisting of whole grains and beans not only interfere with zinc's absorption because of the fiber and phytic acid present in these foods, but also are high in copper, a mineral that is antagonistic to zinc. Zinc and copper ideally should be in an 8:1 ratio in the body; when this ratio is thrown off, numerous conditions such as low immunity, elevated estrogen levels, skin problems, yeast infections, schizophrenia, depression, and lack of mental focus can develop.

The late Carl C. Pfeiffer, Ph.D., M.D., a genius in understanding the roles of nutrients in the body, wrote about this problem: "Zinc insufficiency is one of the greatest and least known dangers of vegetarianism. The individual who does not eat meat must be careful to fulfill the [body's] need for zinc adequately, probably through a tablet supplement. The light-headed feeling of detachment that enshrouds some vegetarians can be caused by hidden zinc hunger, rather than by some mystical quality of the brown rice or other food consumed."

Amino Acid Deficiencies in Vegetarians

Other possible problems vegetarians frequently can develop are deficiencies in several amino acids that animal proteins provide. According to biochemist Don Tyson of Aatron Medical Services, plasma and urine tests reveal that vegetarians commonly are deficient in the amino acids lysine, methionine, tryptophan, carnitine, and taurine. The growing trend for these deficiencies in vegetarians that Tyson sees in his work is alarming, particularly because three of the five amino acids are essential amino acids, which means our body cannot synthesize these in amounts sufficient to meet our physiological needs. Without sufficient amounts of these amino acids, our body can develop numerous ailments ranging from immune system and liver dysfunction to sleep disorders to weight problems.

Just to be on the safe side, to prevent any deficiencies and subsequent health problems from developing, I strongly recommend that all vegetarians have their amino acid profiles tested so they can supplement their diets with any amino acids they may be low in. (See the listing under Aatron Medical Services in the Resources section for more information.)

The Nutritional Pros and Cons of Vegetarianism

As I have discussed, the vegetarian diet carries with it certain risks that haven't been publicized much, making it not suitable for many individuals as a lifelong eating plan. Vegetarianism, however, can be healthy for some individuals who are biologically suited for it, provided they actively plan a balanced diet and make sure they avoid the common nutritional problems vegetarians frequently encounter. They also need to avoid compensating for their lack of animal protein with an excess of carbohydrates or sweet and fatty snack foods. Taking all the pros and cons into account, a vegetarian diet can be effective for many as a short-term therapeutic diet but may not be suitable as a maintenance diet for the majority of Americans.

The History of Meat Eating

Before we consider the choices involved in eating different forms of protein, it might be helpful to consider certain biological and historical facts, many of which I was not aware of when I was stridently vegetarian. I was always told that humans are naturally vegetarian, based on the length of the intestine and the idea that primates are vegetarian (a one-time "fact" now positively disputed by scientific researchers). The long human intestine seems ideal for a fiber-based diet, compared with the short intestine of known carnivores such as dogs. Now I know that this is not the case. History proves that humans have always incorporated meat into their diets. As we've evolved, some individuals have retained a need for more meat in the diet, while others now find they do well on a vegetarian or near-vegetarian diet. The truth is that humans are not basically vegetarian in nature, although many vegetarians—at one time, me included—propose this to be true. According to anthropological researchers S. Boyd Eaton, M.D.,

Marjorie Shostak, and Melvin Konner, Ph.D., authors of *The Pa-leolithic Prescription* (Harper & Row, 1988), paleontological findings clearly support the fact that meat has always been part of the human diet and primate diet.

Exhaustive research into evolution has resulted in the now well-accepted thesis that evolving man has relied on meat as a regular component of the diet *since the beginning*. When the human path diverged from that of the great ape seven million years ago, meat began to assume a *greater* importance in the diet, but had already been part of the primate diet. With the development of stone tools two million years ago, meat became a steady part of the diet.

About 10,000 years ago, the Neolithic Revolution spurred an emphasis on an agricultural life-style because overhunting, climatic changes, and population growth had depleted the meat source to such an extent that fishing, gathering plant foods, and growing grains took on greater importance. Environmental necessity, not biology, spurred the development of domestic grain production. Evolution in the form of physical adaptation to those new foods is still occurring.

Dietary fiber, found in plant foods, also was an important part of the evolving human's diet, and in fact served to aid in the rapid digestion of meat and elimination of waste. Between 20 and 60 percent of our earliest ancestors' dietary calories came from meat, with most groups typically consuming an average of 30 to 35 percent meat in their diets. The rest of their diet was made of leaves, tubers, beans, seeds, nuts, and other plant foods. In addition, our ancestors had a supply of meat that was much lower in saturated fats and higher in the essential fatty acids than the feedlot-raised cattle we now have. Eating free-range chicken, wild game, and beef that are antibiotic- and hormone-free can go a long way in duplicating the proteins of our ancestral diet.

Food Combining for Our Protein Needs?

As I said, proteins serve many necessary functions. They comprise 50 percent of our body's weight. They provide necessary amino acids that cannot be manufactured by the body itself. There are nine essential amino acids, and all of them are contained in animal and fish meat. Vegetable and plant foods have fewer amino acids than meats and thus are considered incomplete proteins. Many vegetarians put a lot of effort into food combining, such as mixing beans with rice, in order to achieve the proper amount of amino acids. There is evidence that such attention to detail may not, in fact, be as helpful as it was once thought. Such a combination may theoretically provide a more complete amino acid combination than when the foods are eaten separately, but may also cause an overload of carbohydrates. As I said in the last chapter, overloading on carbohydrates causes excessive insulin production, conversion of sugar to fat, and an inability to access stored body fat. Even when carefully outlined on paper, combining foods to create enough amino acids doesn't necessarily provide the same nutrition that eating the complete proteins in meat would.

Meatless Not Necessarily Nutritious

There are other problems with a vegetarian diet, including the matter of simply not taking in enough calories. Without dietary balance and moderation among different kinds of foods, vegetarians can develop a sense of gnawing hunger that leads them to fill up not on vegetables but on more fats than are useful to the body. These fats may come from a variety of sources, including fatty dairy products like cheese and yogurt or fatty soy products like tofu and soy milk. They also may rely heavily on carbohydrate-rich foods like granola, rice cakes, and pasta. Then there are the vegetarians I've seen who consider their diet healthy just because it has no meat. Instead, they eat a steady diet of pizza, candy bars, peanut butter sandwiches, fruit, and fruit juices. My observation has been that many of them still struggle with weight problems. All these foods carry their own set of risks. Simply eliminating meat is not the best way to achieve a healthy diet.

Although many people touting a vegetarian diet point to other cultures where meat is of low priority and there is less incidence of the diet-associated health problems that we have in this country, there is simply not enough evidence to finger meat as the culprit. Diets of healthy traditional peoples around the world have been comprised of highly nourishing foods and devoid of junk food and empty calories but have never been totally vegetarian. In addition, it's important once again to remember that a diet that works for one person is not necessarily going to work for another. When considering Third World and traditional diets, you have to take into account ancestry, heritage, blood type, and life-style as well. It is dangerous to superimpose the diets of one culture onto the population of another.

Unlike Third World, Asian, and traditional cultures, Americans typically get 70 percent of their calories from non-nutritious foods. On average, 35 to 40 percent comes from damaged fats like margarine and vegetable oils, 20 percent from refined sugars, and 10 percent from alcohol. Obviously, a reduction in the amount of these foods in our diet is going to be beneficial to our health. Removing meat from the diet is not the answer. Learning to cut back on non-nutritious foods and determining what the right foods are for your own body type is.

The Importance of Balance

This brings me back once again to my ongoing theme, that a diet that may work for some people is not necessarily the best diet for everyone. While some people are able to absorb all the necessary nutrients from a vegetarian diet, others are not. While some people feel clearheaded and energetic on a diet low in animal products, others feel disoriented and sluggish on the same plan. But it's important also to keep in mind the concept of balance. While meat may be necessary for us according to our ancestral diet and the biological needs of our digestive system, it's important to balance its presence in the diet with plenty of fiber in the form of vegetables that are raw or lightly steamed. The vegetables will aid in the digestion of the meat and also provide valuable nutrients that are proven to boost the immune system and fight cancer.

The Spiritual Question of Eating Meat

As conscientious citizens of the world community, many of us have struggled with the spiritual ramifications of eating meat for many years. It has been a long and difficult path, trying to understand the difference between spiritual beliefs and the biological needs of the human body. I certainly don't presume to impose personal beliefs about the "rightness" or "wrongness" of eating meat on anyone, but I do feel it is my duty to present the true facts about the biological and historical presence of meat in the human diet. Please consider: In its most basic form, the human body has a certain program to follow regardless of personal beliefs. And all cultures, even those considered to be highly evolved spiritually, like the traditional Native American culture and the Hindus of India, do incorporate meat into their diet.

The Ayurvedic scriptures, which dictate the traditional Hindu system of medicine, do not teach a vegetarian diet; animals, birds, fish, and mammals all are included in the foods that are to be eaten. In fact, the reason India is primarily vegetarian is not because of a spiritual awakening or for personal health reasons, but because of environmental pressures. It became both uneconomical and unsanitary to raise animals in so crowded an environment.

Dr. Weston Price, in his ground-breaking 20-year research on indigenous and traditional cultures around the world, concluded there were no traditional cultures anywhere that did not place importance on eating animal foods. Oriental cultures include vegetarians and nonvegetarians, but animal foods are thought to contain an energy that other foods do not have and are used to treat certain illnesses that result from a deficiency of the body's basic essence. Native Americans have routinely thanked the animal for giving up its flesh for their nourishment before hunting and eating.

Even *Vegetarian Times* has begun to question whether a vegan diet is right for everyone. A recent article in the magazine explored the different reasons why some former staunch vegetarians have began to add small amounts of meat back to their diet. The article ("Putting Meat Back on Their Menu," *Vegetarian Times,* Jan., 1995, pp. 67–72) quoted Victoria Moran, author of *The Love-Powered Diet* (New World Library, 1992) as saying, "It's a choice" if someone decides to return to eating meat. "They've made one choice [to be a vegetarian]. Now they've made another choice and that's their business."

Personal choice is still exactly that; personal choice. However, I would be remiss if I did not make this point very clear. Whatever personal choice or belief you may have about eating meat, the fact is that the human body has a long history of using some animal protein on a regular basis to thrive. *How* much meat you eat should be determined by your own body type: your family ancestry, your blood type, and your rate of metabolism.

Food for Thought

Have you cut back the fat in your diet so drastically as to have all but eliminated meat, eggs, fish, and poultry? Does knowing more about the beneficial aspects of protein and understanding the misinformation about fat make you feel any more inclined to begin adding these foods to your diet?

Have you made choices about food based on what you thought was right politically, spiritually, or economically? Would the notion that your body chemistry isn't interested in the political agenda of your mind have any impact on your food choices?

Have you feasted on dairy products while excluding eggs from your daily regime? Does knowing that most of us can't utilize the calcium in milk and don't metabolize it without magnesium anyway affect the way you look at dairy advertising?

Would understanding that there is no connection between how many eggs you eat and how high your cholesterol is convince you to start eating eggs again? What if you knew that eating eggs could actually help you lower your cholesterol? It's true. Does this open your eyes to the kind of information whitewash we're all subject to in the popular media?

4

Fat: Essential to the Human Body

Fat is undoubtedly the most maligned nutrient of the century. In fact, I've written entire books about the need for the *right kind* of fats in the diet and the dangers of a no-fat diet. My first book, *Beyond Pritikin,* came out in 1988. Since then, everything I've said about the need for essential fatty acids has been substantiated by dozens of other nutritionists, researchers, and scientists. In fact, the 1990s may well become the Decade of the Essential Fatty Acids.

Fat makes a wonderful source of energy; why do you think our bodies store it so easily? The whole point, if we think back to our earliest ancestors, was to have a stockpile of body energy easily accessible when food supplies dried up. A successful hunt could lead to meat for weeks but was sometimes more the exception than the rule. Besides an erratic supply of game, climatic conditions led to periods when even foraging for food in the form of roots and leaves was difficult. In such situations, the body's store of fat could kick in and be used for energy, not to mention body warmth.

Luckily (or maybe not), our culture no longer has such an erratic food supply. We pretty much have food on demand, and all kinds of food, including proteins, carbohydrates, and fats. We don't have a natural cycle of deprivation to help us use up those fat stores, nor do we maintain nearly the level of physical activity our hunter-gatherer forebears did. In addition, we have been conditioned to believe that eating a lot of bread and pasta instead of meat at meals will not make us fat, when in fact, the opposite is true. If we're eating a lot of carbohydrates, remember, our increased insulin production transforms them into fats, as well as suppresses glucagon, the necessary ingredient for unlocking those stored fat cells to release their energy. The result: We have a lot more body fat than we want, and it's difficult to take off. But the answer is not to eat less fat!

Trans Fats: The Real Villains Causing Our Health Problems

As a culture we consume too much total fat, but it is in the form of vegetable fat (such as processed vegetable oils, margarine, vegetable shortening, and baked goods made from these products). We have been mistakenly led to believe that animal fat was the big problem, but studies prove this isn't so. A study done in Silver Spring, Maryland by Dr. Mary Enig, a leading expert on fats and oils, found that the use of animal fat has markedly *decreased* in the American diet for the past 80 years, falling from 83 percent to 53 percent of total *fat* intake. Conversely, there has been an enormous surge in vegetable fat consumption, from 17 percent in 1910 to 47 percent in 1990. Enig has correlated the rise in vegetable fat consumption with the rise in cancer.

Enig is particularly concerned about vegetable fat in the form of the unnatural trans fats from hydrogenated and partially hydrogenated oils like margarine, vegetable shortening, and soybean oil. Margarine and vegetable shortening are hardened by piping hydrogen through vegetable oils at high temperatures. The hydrogen saturates some of the carbon-carbon bonds of the vegetable oil; this produces a saturated fat. (Margarine is usually not billed as a saturated fat, but it functions like one, due to the processing.)

Although vegetable oil in and of itself has many nutrients, the high temperatures used in converting it into margarine and other hardened forms destroy these nutrients, including the very helpful nutrient vitamin E. Hardening agents also include cadmium and nickel. Nickel is a toxic metal that causes lung and kidney problems when ingested in excess. Cadmium, even more toxic than nickel, has been found to contribute to high blood pressure, cancer, and arteriosclerosis.

In addition, the high-heat processing produces trans fats. While hydrogenated oils may be more stable than unhydrogenated oil (hence their popularity with commercial food producers), the trans fat factor strips the essential fatty acids of their biological potency. Not only can they not be used by the body, their chemical makeup is closer to plastic than to something that would occur in nature!

Foods highest in trans fats are the commercially made baked goods like bread, crackers, rolls, muffins, biscuits, cookies, cakes, pies, and doughnuts. With its long shelf life, partially hydrogenated soybean oil has become a universal favorite for restaurants, manufacturers of processed foods, and fast-food outlets. In 1990, when McDonald's switched from beef tallow to partially hydrogenated vegetable oil for frying their french fries in an attempt to reduce the saturated fat content, the percentage of fat that came from trans fatty acids in their french fries increased from 5 percent to between 42 and 48 percent.

The Detrimental Effects of Trans-Fats

These fats are now considered to be very detrimental to health in a variety of ways. Adverse effects from a diet high in margarine, vegetable shortening, and partially hydrogenated vegetable oils are legion. Cancer, heart disease, obesity, diabetes, and immune system suppression are now associated with the trans fatty acids present in these highly processed and unnatural fats. The structural changes that occur in the fatty acids raise cholesterol and increase the risk of heart disease. The consumption of trans fatty acids *lowers* the level of the protective, or good, HDL cholesterol while *raising* that of the oxidizing, or bad, LDL cholesterol. Consuming foods that contain trans fats actually raises total cholesterol levels more than eating foods with saturated fats.

The process of oxidation is what makes certain fats dangerous elements in the body. Oxidation can occur not only as a natural process of burning energy, but also as part of the processing of foods before they are eaten. Foods become oxidized when they have been left out at room temperature or are smoked, fired, cured, and aged, as sausage, bacon, and cheese are. Dried and powdered egg and milk products, including packaged baking mixes, are also oxidized foods. Processing, packaging, storage, and preparation of foods have a profound effect on oxidation: eating oxidized foods raises your bad LDL cholesterol and lowers the good HDL cholesterol. Oxidation, whether it occurs outside of the body or within as a natural process, also causes the formation of free radicals, which are unstable molecules that alter cell membranes and cellular proteins. Free radicals are pointed to as prime causes of cancer, aging, and heart disease.

Preventing Fats from Causing Harm

By *preventing* the oxidation process from taking place within the body, we can reduce the damage done by oxidative fats. This is where *antioxidants* come in; they prevent the oxidation process from occurring. A diet high in antioxidant-rich foods, such as green and yellow vegetables, can stall or prevent the oxidation process from taking place. Better yet, you can avoid these oxidative fats altogether.

What do you do if you have to give up margarine? Go back to butter! It is a natural source of the fat-soluble vitamins A, D, E, and K. Butter is a partially saturated fat but it is a natural product, not something dreamed up in a chemistry lab, and so is much more acceptable, biologically speaking, to the human body. In *Nutrition and Physical Degeneration,* the landmark book by Dr. Weston Price, butter is identified as having a factor (called "activator X" by Price) that is essential for proper growth and development of bone structure. The best butter you can get (if you don't have your own cow) is made from certified raw cream. It's not widely available, but is worth asking for at your health food store.

This information about trans fats, which I've discussed in more detail in *Beyond Pritikin* and *Super Nutrition for Women,* flies in the face of current nutritional propaganda, which points to meat and animal fat as the dietary culprits responsible for heart disease, obesity, and cancer. Now we know that the artificial and manipulated fats in margarine and hydrogenated and partially hydrogenated vegetable oils are far more dangerous to the human body than the natural fats found in animal meat. Hydrogenation (the manufacturing process of adding hydrogen to oils to solidify them) produces unnatural trans fats that are *biochemically incompatible* with the human body, and have no business being used as food.

Saturated Fat: Good for You?

Aside from these detrimental, man-made fats, there are basically two kinds of natural fats that play a role in human nutrition:

saturated and unsaturated fats. Saturated fats are solid fats found in meats, dairy products like milk and cheese, lard, and beef tallow, as well as tropical oils like coconut and palm kernel oil. A misinformed public has long feared all these saturated fats for their purported link to heart disease.

But, as Dr. Mary Enig states in an interview with biochemist Richard Passwater, Ph.D., (*Whole Foods,* December, 1993): "The idea that saturated fats cause heart disease is completely wrong, but the statement has been 'published' so many times over the last three or more decades that it is very difficult to convince people otherwise unless they are willing to take the time to read and learn what all the economic and political factors were that produced the anti-saturated fat agenda. . . . The latest theories regarding heart disease point to oxidized fats and oxidized lipoproteins as culprits. This being the case, accusations against chemically stable, basically nonoxidizable saturated fat don't make sense. Most people who find fault with saturated fats do not really understand that our cells are busy making saturated fatty acids all the time from carbohydrates and excess protein."

I agree with Dr. Enig but only to a point as I will explain in a moment. The reason I quote her to such an extent is because saturated fats, just like red meat and eggs, have been vilified in the press as dangerous foods that must be banished from everyone's diet, something I definitely don't agree with. Saturated fats play a positive role in the human body. They provide a good source of stored energy, they cushion the organs against shock, and they insulate vital tissues against the cold. The body's capacity for energy storage in the form of fat cells is an evolutionary marvel. Over millions of years our bodies have adapted to periodic famine by building up an energy reserve. Nature in her wisdom provides extra protection for women for childbearing and nursing by storing extra reserves (fat) in the buttocks, thighs, and breasts.

When Are Saturated Fats Harmful?

There are problems associated with saturated fats in the diet, but they are related more to excessive consumption and to the lack of the regulating EFAs. The prime sources of saturated fats in our diet are fast foods and foods that are frozen or processed, such as convenience foods and frozen meals. We tend to overeat saturated fats not because we are eating too many fresh, thick steaks but because we unwittingly eat fats that are separated from the original food sources and used in a variety of ways in commercial food production. Beef tallow, tropical oils, and vegetable oils are used for fast-food production, especially for deep-fat frying, and are added to milkshakes and nondairy creamers. If you're like the average American, you eat out at restaurants (including fast-food chains) for more than one third of your meals; that can add up to a lot of hidden saturated fat you weren't counting on. And if you have a freezer stuffed with quick meals you can just pop in the microwave, you're getting a lot more hidden fat. The average frozen food entree contains over 50 percent fat. (The low-fat versions are remarkably high in carbohydrates, which is almost as bad, as I've discussed earlier.)

Overindulging in saturated fats—unwittingly or not—can affect your health. Saturated fats can block the conversion of the good fats—essential fatty acids—into beneficial prostaglandins. Prostaglandins are tissuelike hormones that are vital in regulating the cardiovascular system as well as the reproductive, immune, and central nervous systems. Prostaglandins also have been shown to lower blood cholesterol and triglycerides and to promote overall cardiovascular protection by inhibiting blood clots, dilating blood vessels, and lowering blood pressure. Indirectly, overconsumption of saturated fats promotes heart disease by blocking the formation of these beneficial prostaglandins.

Avoiding the Dangers of Saturated Fats

There are two ways to increase the amount of meat (and protein) in your diet—something I believe many of the low-fat diet proponents need to do—without succumbing to the dangers of saturated fats. One is to avoid highly processed and frozen foods like frozen dinners, and to cut down on the number of trips you make to fast-food chains, diners, and other restaurants where a lot of the cooking is done with saturated fats. The other is to eat meat from range-fed cattle, which is very high in essential fatty acids, rather than feedlot cattle. Meat from cattle raised on feedlots is well-marbled with exactly the wrong kind of fat. Instead of being high in the good, essential fatty acids like meat from their range-fed cousins, feedlot cattle meat is very high in saturated fat.

Small amounts of saturated fat as part of a well-balanced diet that is geared specifically to your own metabolic type should not be considered a problem. What is more dangerous to the body than saturated fats—which are, as I've pointed out, manufactured naturally in the human body—is the lack of the good fats—essential fatty acids. I'll be discussing EFAs later in this chapter.

Also, keep in mind my discussion about cholesterol in the previous chapter on proteins. It is not necessary to avoid cholesterol-containing foods. Only about 4 percent of all cholesterol comes from the diet anyway, no matter how much you eat. The rest is manufactured in the body. And a major cause of a high cholesterol level in our body is stress. In stressful times, the body responds by manufacturing more cholesterol, which can then be converted into the adrenal hormones the body uses to handle stress. Reducing stress—emotional or biochemical—can bring about a decrease in your cholesterol level.

In answer to whether tropical oils, which are the saturated fats that were so diligently removed from commercially produced cookies and crackers a short while back, are harmful, Enig has this to say: "Several studies have shown that there is no increase in heart disease in countries or communities where most of the fat is either coconut oil or palm oil. Palm oil that is not extensively refined has very high levels of antioxidants, and coconut oil has high levels of very useful medium-chain fatty acids. There are many older research studies that showed that adding quite a bit of coconut oil to the diets of persons having high blood cholesterol reduced their level of cholesterol. Dr. George Blackburn, from Harvard Medical School, has written an extensive review on this topic.

"It is unfortunate that this misinformation about these oils became so widespread because they are very stable oils that have unique functional properties and products made with them as a fat component usually have far less fat and fewer calories. Needless to say, they would also have virtually no trans fatty acids, which are unquestionably atherogenic. When coconut oil was used in the manufacture of crackers, very little fat was added to each cracker, and the crackers did not become stale before they could be purchased. Now the fat-free crackers become very stale very quickly and the crackers made with more unsaturated oils are higher in fat and are greasy or they appear drier because they are made with high-temperature-melting partially hydrogenated oils. Deep fried foods made in these oils never absorb quite as much fat as they do when they are made with the more unsaturated oils."

This aspect of Dr. Enig's discussion is something I fully agree with. As she said, the healthiest versions of tropical oils like palm and coconut are in a mostly unrefined state, but even as an ingredient in processed foods like crackers, they are a much better choice than the alternative, the dreaded hydrogenated oils and trans fats.

However, going back to my earlier discussion about carbohydrates, I frankly don't find a whole lot of room in a healthy, slimming diet for crackers! Not because of the kinds of oils that may have been used in the processing, but because they are a carbohydrate that causes a rise in insulin and blocks production of your fat-burning resource, glucagon.

Eating Fat to Lose Fat

In addition to the reasons I listed earlier, there is another important reason that fat should be included in the diet. Fat levels out blood sugar. As a slow-burning nutrient, fat actually slows down the release of carbohydrate into your system and improves the ratio of insulin to glucagon, essential for mobilizing stored body fat out of the body. That's right, some fat in the diet is necessary to assist the process of burning off stored fat! Unlike carbohydrates, which can create food cravings, fat can also keep your appetite satisfied for up to six hours at a time, protecting you from the temptations of sugary snacks.

The French Paradox

Consider the French Paradox: France has a much lower rate of heart disease than America, but the diet there is heavy in saturated fats. American men have an average cholesterol reading of 209 milligrams and a cardiovascular disease death rate of 197 per 100,000. The French cholesterol level averages 230 milligrams per deciliter but their death rate is only 78 per 100,000.

In France, people eat four times as much butter, twice as much cheese, and the same number of calories that we consume. They eat twice as much animal fat and only two thirds the amount of vegetable oils in the American diet. The French eat only one eighteenth (5 percent) of the sugar consumed in this country, but more vegetables, more fish, more whole grains, more potatoes, and more of other complex carbohydrates. They also consume half the amount of fruit Americans do, and they do not snack in between meals.

How can the saturated fat be the culprit in our diets when the French eat so much more than we do and do not have the same degenerative diseases we do? Research indicates that the American diet, which is high in *artificial fats* and *sugar,* may be more dangerous than a diet high in natural fats and very low in sugar, like the French diet. In addition, the French are big believers in fresh foods, whereas Americans are conditioned for convenience and often opt for packaged, processed, frozen, and canned foods, which may contain hidden sugars as well as being stripped of their nutrients and being high in chemicals and preservatives. It may well be that the emphasis on increased consumption of potatoes, fresh vegetables, and red wine in the French diet provides antioxidants, which stop fat from oxidizing in the body.

The incidence of heart attacks in America has not gone down even though consumption of saturated fats and cholesterol levels have. I believe the reason fewer deaths are resulting from heart attacks is due more to medical technology and improved intervention techniques (bypass, angioplasty, and angiograms) than to the promotion of the low-fat diet.

The Roles of Unsaturated Fats and Essential Fatty Acids

In addition to saturated fats, we need to consider unsaturated fats for their important components—essential fatty acids. Unsaturated fats are the fats found in vegetable, seed, nut, and fish oils and are divided into two categories: monounsaturated fats and polyunsaturated fats. Monounsaturated fats are found in canola oil, olives and olive oil, avocados, peanuts, almonds, and cashews. Polyunsaturated fats are found in fish (salmon, mackerel, halibut), vegetable oils (corn, safflower, sunflower, sesame) and botanicals (borage and evening primrose).

The important aspect of polyunsaturated oils is that they contain **essential fatty acids** (once known as vitamin F), which are vital to the integrity of the cell membrane, the first defense against bacterial and viral infections. Without essential fats, the cell membrane becomes weakened, and viral infections have easy access to the body's systems. Surprisingly, *eating fat can help you become thin*, because EFAs also move other fats, including the bad LDL cholesterol, out of the body. They emulsify and move saturated fats and cholesterol through the bloodstream and out of artery and tissue deposits. This is especially beneficial for liquefying and eliminating the stored hard fats of overweight individuals.

There are two major types of essential fatty acids: **omega-3 oils** from flax seed, walnut, chia, canola, pumpkin seed oils, and cold-water fatty fish like salmon, mackerel, sardine, tuna, and anchovy; and **omega-6 oils** found in plant sources such as unprocessed, unheated vegetable oils including safflower, sunflower, corn, and sesame, as well as botanicals like borage and evening primrose. (Some EFAs are also present in saturated animal fat, but I recommend seeking out free-range, chemical-free meats because they have a much greater presence of EFAs than feedlot and grain-fed meats.) These EFA's are quickly taken into the cell membranes rather than stored as padding, and they also are burned up in the body faster than most other dietary fats.

EFAs also produce prostaglandins, which regulate our cardiovascular, immune, endocrine, central nervous, digestive, and reproductive systems. In short, all the systems of our body depend on the presence of EFAs. A deficiency in EFAs can cause dry, flaky skin, inflammation, arthritis, acne, eczema, and a variety of other symptoms.

Something that most people don't realize is that cholesterol molecules attach to EFAs to move through the bloodstream. If the

EFAs are not available, then the cholesterol latches on to saturated fat molecules instead, and ends up coating the arteries. That's why getting enough essential fatty acids is so important in helping lower cholesterol and reduce the risk of heart disease.

Depending on your biological nutritional needs, you may not need to limit your consumption of saturated fats, as some biochemical types rely on a higher amount of fat in the diet. *Fast burners* generally can eat more butter and fatty foods, and usually have lower cholesterol levels than slow burners. They slow burn up the fat they eat rapidly and efficiently. *Slow burners* are better off restricting fats and oils to a specific daily amount, as you'll see in Chapter 9, where I discuss what to eat.

To protect oneself against coronary artery disease and other degenerative diseases, everyone should totally avoid margarine, vegetable shortening, and partially hydrogenated vegetable oils. But you **cannot** eliminate the EFAs (found in flaxseed oil, safflower oil, canola oil, linseed oil, evening primrose oil, and, as omega-3, in fish) without doing damage to your system.

The Hazards of Too Little Fat

In our mania to cut fat out of our diets, some people have gone too far. In my practice, I frequently see clients who, in their misguided quest to eliminate all fat, do not get a daily supply of EFAs. Their health suffers for it and, to top it off, they don't lose weight. EFAs are necessary to help you lose weight, and incidentally can also alleviate PMS problems. One EFA in particular, GLA (gamma linolenic acid, found in evening primrose oil), specifically activates the fat-burning process in the body, but my first experience with it was to prescribe it to my clients to smooth out difficult menstrual periods.

A Rule of Thumb for EFAs

As with carbohydrates and proteins, there is no one standard amount of essential fatty acids that works for everybody all the time. People seem to need differing amounts of EFAs. As a general rule of thumb, however, I like to suggest at least 1 tablespoon of flaxseed oil a day for the omega-3 it provides and 1 tablespoon of unprocessed safflower oil or four capsules of GLA or evening primrose oil for the omega-6 they supply. This should provide the necessary amount of EFAs to keep your cells burning off fat as well as all the other benefits I've mentioned. (An in-depth discussion of EFAs and the role they play in weight loss and optimal health can be found in my books *Beyond Pritikin, Super Nutrition for Women,* and *Super Nutrition for Menopause.*)

Differences in EFA and Fat Needs

Remember that the suggestion to take 1 tablespoon of flax oil and 1 tablespoon of safflower oil each day is just a rule of thumb. The suggestion might not work for everyone because we each have vastly different genetic makeups that cause us to handle some fats better than others. One concept that can help us determine which fats may be best for us is the understanding of "northern" and "southern" oils.

In order to know which kinds of oils may be genetically right for us, we first need to remember that heat and light (including sunlight) damage fats, and they damage polyunsaturated fats more than saturated ones. In an amazing adaptation to the sunlight and heat present in each area of the world, nature has caused plants, animals, and humans that develop in the tropics to contain more saturated fatty acids in their fat tissue than the same plants, animals, and humans that grow in polar regions.

What this means to you and me is that if your ancestors came from Africa, Polynesia, or any other area of the tropics, you are genetically programmed to be more able to handle saturated fats like those found in coconut and palm oils (what I call southern oils). If your heritage is from the Mediterranean area, you probably have more of an affinity for monounsaturated fats like those found in olive and almond oils, whereas people with ancestors from temperate zones do well with different forms of polyunsaturated oils, like safflower and sunflower. Those with ancestors from the polar regions of the earth thrive on large amounts of highly unsaturated fatty acids, especially omega-3 essential fatty acids like those found in flaxseed oil and cold-water fish oils. (These types of oils are often referred to as northern oils.)

Since most of us are blends of several different nationalities, it's not as easy for us to determine the types of oils and fats we should consume as it is for the person who has ancestral roots from one distinct area. Understanding the concept of northern and southern oils, however, gives us important clues about the oils and foods that may be most beneficial for us. Remember to listen to the messages your body gives you as you continue to personalize your diet.

Don't Feel Guilty about Eating Some Fat

Now that I have reintroduced you to the value of proteins, fats, and carbohydrates in the diet, it is my hope that no one will feel guilty about eating some meat and fat again. In the next chapter, I am going to take a brief look at several diet plans that have recently become popular. Armed with your new understanding about fats, carbohydrates, and proteins, you'll see how these diets are supposed to work and why they don't.

Food for Thought

Let's say you have the choice of butter or margarine for your slice of whole-grain toast. Do you choose the one that is a natural product and a good source of several vitamins? Or do you choose the one that advertisers have conditioned us to believe is better for your health, the one that has been created in a chemistry lab, the one that has been stripped of any of its naturally occurring nutrients, the one that has been so chemically altered during processing that it is virtually incompatible with the human body?

Did you give up your favorite crackers because they were made with tropical oils? Were you thrilled that they came back on the market with fresh new labels stating "No Tropical Oils" and "Low Fat"? Do you understand now why you should avoid them, and why it has nothing to do with the oil?

In your efforts to eat a low-fat diet, have you found yourself eliminating foods that contain the very fats your body needs and depends on for a strong, slender body and good health? For a week or two, maybe you could try changing nothing in your diet except adding 2 tablespoons a day of flaxseed or safflower oil, or four evening primrose oil capsules, and see if your body changes.

5

What's Wrong with Current Diet Trends?

With our new understanding of how carbohydrates, fats, and proteins work in the body, let's now take a brief look at the most popular diets to see how they compare. The main feature of many popular diets is that they favor one nutrient over others: some contain an abundance of carbohydrates, whereas others are higher in protein or fat. Most of these plans generally have an abysmal success rate for one specific reason: they only work for certain people whose metabolism and ancestral type can accommodate a diet that emphasizes one type of food to the exclusion of others. People who need more protein do not do well at all on high-carbohydrate diets, vegetarian diets, or diets in which fruit is a main component. And for the people with a metabolism that can handle large amounts of carbohydrates without increased insulin production, introducing a lot of protein into the diet can really slow them down.

Remember: What works for one person is not necessarily going to work for another. The key is understanding your metabolism, blood type, and ancestry and the foods that will work best for you.

Here's a review of the current popular diets and why they help some people and don't help others:

Calorie-Restrictive Diets

These include diets prescribing fewer than 1,000 calories and meal-replacement diets such as Slim-Fast. We used to think there were basically only two ways to lose weight: burn more calories with exercise or take in fewer calories with diet. While exercise is still one of the best ways to activate your metabolism, calorie counting is not, and never has been, an effective way to lose weight. In fact, contrary to what you may have been hearing all these years, reducing calories, your body's fuel, is a sure way to hold on to your body fat. If you suddenly drop the amount of calories your body is used to consuming, your body will assume you are in a famine situation and will immediately slow down your metabolism (your calorie-burning rate) in order to keep what energy stores you have. Skipping meals actually lowers the metabolic rate. Simply eating your basic three meals a day can burn up to 10 percent more calories than are used skipping any one of them.

A slowing of your metabolism halts weight loss. We make less thyroid hormone on low-calorie diets in an effort to conserve calories and, as a result, the body actually becomes more efficient at storing fat. You might call this the starvation response, because our bodies can't tell the difference between true famine and a self-imposed calorie-restricted diet. Once the calorie supply is cut, the enzyme lipase becomes more active in preparing fat to be stored in fat cells, where it can be accessed as an energy source if the "famine" continues. Lipase activity may increase 25-fold in low-calorie repeat dieters.

Repeated calorie cutting also leads to the notorious yo-yo dieting syndrome. This refers to cycles of weight gain and loss from a nonstop succession of dieting, something you probably are familiar with. There are many documented hazards that result from yo-yo dieting. Body fat may be redistributed from thighs and hips to the abdomen. The fatter we are from the waist up, the greater the risk we run of contracting for diabetes and heart disease ('tis better to be a pear than an apple!). Yo-yo dieting may also increase the body's fat-to-lean tissue ratio. Muscle tissue may be lost while dieting, but when weight is regained, it is always in the form of fat.

If you start an intense exercise program in tandem with a severe calorie-cutting diet, you will have even less energy to burn off in strenuous activity than you did before you started dieting. You want to burn off the fat you already have, not the fuel you're eating every day for your body's building blocks. Exercise is an important component of weight loss and, as I discuss in Chapter 7, it is much more effective than calorie cutting. If you only do one thing to lose weight, it should be adding exercise, *not* reducing your calorie intake.

One of the biggest problems with extremely low calorie diets is that dieters develop such a fear of food that they barely eat all day. By late afternoon or evening, these poor dieters are literally starving, and begin to binge on whatever foods may be available. Emotional stress from such a diet and the resulting guilty feelings can lead to serious eating disorders like anorexia and bulimia, in addition to contributing to a never-ending cycle of weight loss and gain.

Nutritionally speaking, people are confused about calories. Obesity is on the rise for two calorie-connected reasons. 1) We eat a lot of high-calorie foods that are excessively high in sugar and fat, and low in vitamins, minerals, and other nutrients like protein. Some of these foods include ice cream, chocolate bars, croissants, and muffins. 2) We also eat low-calorie foods in our mania to avoid fat, foods like pasta, breads, crackers, and cereals. These foods do not satisfy our hunger or our vital nutritional needs; they are not vitamin-or mineral-rich, and our bodies burn them so quickly that they don't provide long-lasting energy.

Excessive amounts of high-calorie foods (like desserts or fatty fast-food meals) that have little to offer in the way of a long-term energy source are called empty calories. We are much better off eating a high-calorie food like a steak (protein) with lots of vegetables (complex carbohydrate, fiber), a little canola oil (EFA), and some steamed brown rice (complex carbohydrate, fiber) than a big plate of pasta (low-calorie processed carbohydrate) with a creamy cheese sauce (high-calorie fat) and bread (processed carbohydrate).

You may eat more calories in the steak than in the pasta, but the steak offers the necessary building component of protein and its amino acids, as well as fat to slow digestion enough to maintain a steady stream of energy rather than the instant rush pasta affords. The result of eating steak is actually more internal assistance in accessing stored fat, more energy for fat-burning exercise, and the building of stronger tissues, muscles, and bones.

The Low-Fat, High-Carbohydrate Diet

Variations of the low-fat, high-carbo diet are probably the most widespread these days. They include diets by Pritikin, Ornish, McDougall, and others. The Rice Diet is an example of this type of diet in its most extreme form. Also referred to by the popular generic "light diet," this regimen emphasizes carbohydrates (primarily in the form of whole grains, breads, and pastas as well as legumes, fruits, and vegetables), skinless chicken and lean fish, and a very low intake of fat. Some of these diets are vegetarian. This means not only low or no intake of lean meats and nonfat dairy products but also of oils, which could contain EFA's. Some people thrive on this diet; others suffer. Why doesn't it work for everyone?

There are two main reasons: the insulin connection and a sensitivity to gluten. As I have discussed, overconsumption of carbohydrates leads to overproduction of insulin, which converts blood sugar to body fat and suppresses glucagon, which otherwise would release stored body fat for energy. This diet causes constant hunger cravings and fatigue because of the low amount of protein and fat included. Hunger cravings (and low-calorie intake) lead to perpetual snacking, especially on fruit, "natural" cookies sweetened with fruit juice, and high-glycemic foods such as rice cakes. With the emphasis on grains, gluten is much more prevalent in the diet and, in combination with a low level of EFA's and body-building protein, a diet like this can cause a host of symptoms to occur, from yeast infections and PMS to chronic fatigue syndrome, loss of hair, flaky skin, and lack of stamina and endurance.

This diet is especially detrimental to the *fast burner* and the person with blood type O, both of whom need protein on a regular basis. *Slow burners* and A blood types do much better on this sort of diet, although slow burners need more protein than is usually recommended on a high-carbohydrate, low-fat diet like this.

Liquid Low- or No-Carbohydrate, Low-Fat, High-Protein Diets

These diets rely on protein powders and liquid protein fasts (for example, Optifast) and often restrict carbohydrates. Without some carbohydrates to maintain blood sugar levels and fuel the system, ketone bodies—fatty substances generated from the breakdown of stored fats or triglycerides—are soon formed in the blood. Ketone bodies mask your appetite even though your brain demands glucose. The result is ketosis: headaches, light-headedness, and mental fatigue. Eventually your body will begin to convert protein from your muscles into blood sugar. You lose weight, but it is from muscle mass, not from fat. You also lose a lot of water weight on a diet like this because your body excretes large amounts of water to remove the ketones and excess nitrogen. This process stresses the kidneys and liver. Electrolyte depletion is also a hazard. Once you go off the diet, you gain the weight back, but not as muscle mass. You gain back fat.

Furthermore, the lack of fiber in these diets impedes proper movement of toxins from the bowels out of the body. In addition, fructose is often the sweetener of choice in liquid diet shakes. Please see my discussion of pages 98–100 about diets high in fructose.

An excessive intake of protein also causes a depletion of cal-cium stores, resulting in brittle bones and osteoporosis. Other possible damaging effects include kidney stones and renal failure, stress on the liver and kidneys, and increased uric acid levels and risk of gout. Once again, the idea of the balanced diet, in which all the components necessary to insure healthy body functions are introduced to the body through a variety of foods in proportion, starts to make sense.

High-Protein, Low-Carbohydrate Diets

The Atkins diet, Scarsdale diet, Carbohydrate Addict's diet, Stillman diet, and the Endocrine Control Diet are all high-protein, low-carbohydrate diets. These plans primarily work for *fast-burners* (people who metabolize food into fuel quickly) who need the higher protein and fat content to slow down their overactive metabolisms. *Slow burners* have a disastrous response to these diets because their specific metabolism requires more carbohydrates than are found in this limited-carbohydrate program. Fast burners are able to utilize the high amount of fats in these diets for energy, but slow burners are not; instead, the fat just slows them down even more and is more easily converted to body fat. In addition, the reduced carbohydrate content of these diets in the form of legumes and grains can result in constipation.

Macrobiotic Diet

This diet based on a carefully formulated balance of certain foods has been heavily promoted as a cancer-controlling diet. Although one can incorporate endless modifications, the basic macrobiotic diet is approximately 50 percent or more whole grains, 25 percent land and sea vegetables, 10 to 15 percent beans and bean products, and 15 percent or less animal foods. Small amounts of nuts, seeds, and fruits can also be added. An important facet of the macrobiotic diet is the emphasis on eating foods that are in season, such as squash, root vegetables, turnips, and parsnips in the fall and fresh fruits and salad vegetables in the summer. Many cancer patients give enthusiastic testimonials about the healing properties of this diet. Like the Ornish plan, it can be very effective as a therapeutic diet. However, it is not always suitable for a maintenance dietary regimen, as I explained in the example of James Templeton (in this book's Introduction).

Fast burners would not be adequately nourished on the macrobiotic diet because of the lack of high-fat and high-purine protein foods like red meat, organ meats, sardines, and herring. *Slow burners,* on the other hand, will fare much better, as long as lean proteins are included on a daily basis. However, the high sodium content in many of the condiments (sea salt, tamari, miso, soy sauce) can cause high blood pressure, water retention, and muscular tightness if the condiments are used in excess, which is a common occurrence due to the blandness of the foods. In addition, the mostly soy-based condiments used in the macrobiotic diet are not tolerated well by the majority of Americans. Many food allergists rank soy high on the list of items that cause allergic reactions. Although soy is a food that has a long history of use among people of Oriental heritage, it has not been used extensively by people of other nationalities. Finally, James and I have observed that there seems to be a lot of cigarette smoking and coffee drinking among those who follow a strict macrobiotic diet. We've concluded that the caffeine and nicotine are used as energy stimulants to those on this nutrient-deficient diet.

Fruit and Juicing Diets

The most popular fruit-based diets, including the Beverly Hills, Fit for Life, and Juiceman diets, emphasize heavy consumption of fruit during much of the day and fruit and vegetable juices accompanying every meal or replacing meals. All of that fruit can damage the body. It is suggested that the high water content of fruits and vegetables makes them ideal diet and detoxification foods, but the high sugar level in the form of fructose is not taken into account by those who recommend this kind of regimen.

Remember my earlier discussion on fructose? Fructose is a simple sugar that converts very easily into glucose (starting off the production of insulin, which blocks the production of fat-burning glucagon) and is especially known for *stimulating fat storage!* Fructose also goes directly to the liver, where it is converted to triglycerides, a fat that raises the risk of heart attack.

In addition, although many individuals think that fruit juices couldn't begin to cause the problems that other sugars cause, large quantities of fruit juice do wreak havoc with blood sugar functioning. Erratic blood sugar levels frequently lead to food bingeing during low blood sugar episodes, helping to cause weight gain instead of weight loss.

Many of my clients who eat a lot of fruit, fruit juices, and fruit-juice sweetened snacks have not been able to lose weight until I limited them to one to two pieces of fresh fruit a day and eliminated all fruit juices and fruit-juice-sweetened snacks from their diets. Not only can excessive fructose make you fat, but it can also inhibit the synthesis of protein and actually impair your immune system. Ingesting the amount of sugar (fructose) in a glass of orange juice depresses the immune system by 50 percent within two hours, an effect that can last for several hours.

The hunger mechanism and the thirst mechanism are two different activities in the body; they have different needs and are satisfied in different ways. When you are thirsty, your body's requesting water, which makes up over 70 percent of the human body. When you are hungry, your body is asking for food: calories, protein, fat, and carbohydrates are needed for all the various functions of the complicated machinery of the body. Converting fruits and vegetables (food) into juices and drinking them instead of drinking water confuses both your hunger and your thirst mechanisms. The end result is that neither is satisfied.

This diet is also very low in animal protein, verging on the vegetarian, which is a suitable diet only for certain metabolic types. Once again the dieter faces a lack of protein, the essential building block of the body, as well as a lack of calories, which can lead to snacking on high-fat and sugary foods. In fact, most of these diets recommend a low daily calorie intake as well as an increase in physical activity. The result is that not enough calories are taken in to maintain increased exertion levels and you are left feeling exhausted. You run out of steam and don't have enough energy even for ordinary tasks, let alone a daily aerobics class or run. To compensate, you try to fill up on carbohydrates like bread, pasta, bagels, or sweets, hoping to get a quick energy rush from the sugar. You already know what that means: increased insulin production and suppressed glucagon production, conversion of sugars to body fat and no access to already-stored fat for energy.

Finally, you may enter such a cycle of carbohydrate dependence just to provide enough energy to get through the day that you could burn out your endocrine system, the glands that provide necessary energy sources like adrenaline. You wind up chronically fatigued, vulnerable to germs and sickness, and yet still not necessarily any slimmer than when you started.

Cleansing Diet

The Burroughs Diet, Three-Day Fast, and Liver Flush are examples of cleansing diets. Promoted primarily as a healing diet used in the prevention of treatment of illness, the cleansing diet serves an important purpose but should not be considered a maintenance diet. Effective for clearing out toxins from the colon and intestines, the cleansing diet, which may be exclusively fruit and vegetable juice or may contain whole grains and vegetables but no protein, does not provide enough nutrients for a long-standing dietary regimen. After experiencing an initial period of weight loss and a sense of well-being, the person on this sort of dietary regimen will begin to feel exhausted and undernourished. Research has shown that after two or three days on a strict cleansing diet, enzymes in the liver responsible for detoxification cease to function effectively. The elements you are trying to eliminate from your body then actually are converted into something worse. Incomplete detoxification is worse than no detoxification, because if the process is not completed, you have a more potent, toxic compound in your body than what you started with.

For people who wish to periodically engage in a short-term cleansing diet in order to rid their bodies of metabolic wastes, chemicals, and allergens, I recommend a product called the Fat Flush Kit (It can be ordered by calling 1-800-888-4353). It can be used by itself or in conjunction with a special cleansing diet. The benefits of the Fat Flush Kit are many: 1) it may improve the liver detoxification response, 2) it is totally vegetarian and can be used even in a vegan diet is necessary, and 3) it may improve the body's capacity to respond to toxins in the future.

Food for Thought

Have you always thought if you just ate less food—hence, less calories—that you would lose weight? And if you ate less food and exercised more, you would do even better? Do you see now why that has always led to yo-yo dieting in the past? Do you pledge never to return to a calorie-cutting diet again as a way to lose weight?

•

Has juicing seemed an appealing way to lose weight? Have you noticed how hungry you get when you eat nothing but juiced vegetables?

•

It seems almost too good to be true, that you could get all the nutrition you need to help you lose weight in a can filled with a chocolate milkshake. It is too good to be true. You don't get the nutrients you need, you don't lose weight, and you could be endangering your health.

•

Look around at the people you work with, the people you socialize with. Can you imagine what would happen if all of them went on the same dietary regime? Could it be true, that there is no one diet that works for everyone?

6

Determining Your Type
and Putting
Your Diet Together

W hat all this information boils down to is whether you should be eating a diet that relies heavily on carbohydrates or one that calls for increased protein and fat. You can determine which route is best for you based on whether you are a *fast* or *slow burner* and what your blood type and ancestry are.

For fast burners, a diet that is weighted toward protein and fat with fewer carbohydrates is the best one to provide sustained energy. Slow burners should eat less fat and more carbohydrates and protein in order to speed up the metabolism and burn existing fat stores. Processed carbohydrates like bread, pasta, bagels, muffins, and crackers are not recommended for *either* type, and should be kept to a minimum. In fact, the only people who can really do well on a diet that is high in these carbohydrates are people who are extremely physically active, like athletes, and aerobics teachers. Even if you work out every day, unless it's for several hours at a time, there's no way you'll be utilizing all the energy provided by those carbs; it just turns into fat. And keep in mind that many athletes have also found that adding protein to their high-carbohydrate diet actually boosted their energy level and helped them burn off stored body fat.

The only thing left to do is determine your metabolic type, which is not such a difficult thing if you are at all on speaking terms with your body. Once you determine whether you are a fast or slow burner, you can modify your diet based upon your blood type and ancestral heritage. Determining your metabolic type is really the most important factor when customizing your diet. Rate of metabolism dominates *how* the body is utilizing whatever foods you eat and, in most cases, should take precedence over blood type and ancestry when determining the right diet for yourself.

By the way, it's true that there are people who are neither fast nor slow burners, but whose metabolic rate falls right in the middle. Those people rarely struggle with weight problems because their bodies are using up food at just the right speed to keep them healthy and slim. They've also probably managed to latch on to just the right combination of foods to eat to keep their motors humming along without a glitch, feeling neither edgy and hyper nor sluggish and slow. If you're experiencing a weight problem or any of the other health symptoms I've discussed, then looking into the metabolism factor is one of the most important things you can do for yourself.

Blood type and ancestry are modifying factors that should be considered on a secondary basis. There's no denying their importance, as we've seen, but they still play second fiddle to how quickly your body is able to use the food you eat.

What's Your Type?

How do you know if you are a *fast* or *slow burner*? You need to listen to your own body. It will give you all the information you need to determine if your metabolism tends towards the fast or slow.

Here are two questionnaires that will help you better define whether you are a slow burner or a fast burner or somewhere in between. If you find that a certain characteristic applies to you only some of the time, consider that you may fall into the range between fast and slow, which means your metabolism may be at a good balance. Those who do fall in between would benefit from a more balanced approach to diet than one that is more weighted to one type of food or another. Remember, I am asking about general tendencies in the following questionnaires. No one is necessarily one way all of the time. If a question asks about something that you experience more often than not, it should be answered yes.

Slow Burner Questionnaire

1. Are you somewhat laid back and even-tempered? yes ___ no ___

2. Does red meat feel heavy in your system? yes ___ no ___

3. Do you approach problems one step at a time, rather than juggling many things at once? yes ___ no ___

4. Can you skip breakfast without losing energy or getting hungry? yes ___ no ___

5. Do sweet things like candy or fruit give you a quick pickup? yes ___ no ___

6. Do you prefer a "light" meal of salad pasta to a "heavier" one of steak and potato? yes ___ no ___

7. Do you get thirsty a lot? yes ___ no ___

8. Do foods like cheese, butter, and avocados seem to make you sluggish? yes ___ no ___

9. Does coffee start your morning off just right? yes ___ no ___

10. Do you feel you need a pick-up from spices and particularly enjoy tangy condiments like mustard, ketchup, and salsa with your food? yes ___ no ___

Scoring the Slow Burner Questionnaire

If you answered yes to eight or more of these questions, you are a classic *slow burner* type. The best way to approach a healthy eating plan is to incorporate the following guidelines into your eating habits:

- A slow burner should maintain a diet that is *lighter on fatty foods and heavier on both complex (not processed) carbohydrates and protein.* You'll find a complete guide to the proper foods and a list of menus for slow burners in Chapter 9.
- If you are a slow burner, make sure to include lean protein in *two meals a day* because it will speed up your metabolism and counteract the reduced rate of energy release you experience from the carbohydrates you eat.
- Avoid fatty meats like ribs and steaks, and dairy products like milk and cheese in favor of *poultry, eggs, and light fish,* like cod and tuna.
- Keep in mind my warnings about excessive processed carbohydrate consumption. Eat *vegetables and whole grains* (in addition to lean meats) but avoid processed carbohydrates like bread, bagels, pasta, crackers, etc.

You may already be eating a low-fat diet, but if you are not eating enough protein, your system will remain too slow to effectively burn off fat stores and provide continuous energy throughout the day. Protein is a vital component of the slow burner's optimal diet, but should be taken from lean proteins like fish and fowl rather than the heartier meats like beef and lamb. A vegetarian diet is not suitable for the slow burner because protein is an essential component in speeding up a sluggish metabolism and helping to release stored fat for energy.

If you answered yes to five to seven questions, you tend toward being a slow burner, and the recommendations for the slow burner diet still apply to you at least three to four days a week or two meals a day. If you answered no to most of these questions, then look ahead to the next questionnaire, because you may be a fast burner instead.

Fast Burner Questionnaire

1. Do you consider yourself high strung, or feel hyperactive? yes ___ no ___

2. Do you actually feel better eating a plate of chops rather than leaner meats like chicken? yes ___ no ___

3. Do you enjoy a hearty high-protein breakfast (eggs and bacon)? yes ___ no ___

4. Do you reach for salty snacks like nuts or potato chips when you are stressed out? yes ___ no ___

5. Are avocado, cheesy sauces, and full-fat dairy products very satisfying to you? yes ___ no ___

6. Do you feel better eating full meals every two to three hours? yes ___ no ___

7. When you eat sweet foods like cakes and cookies, do you burn out quickly after a short energy burst? yes ___ no ___

8. Do you have a hearty appetite? yes ___ no ___

9. Does drinking coffee make you nervous? yes ___ no ___

10. Does a pat of butter on toast satisfy you more than jam?
yes ___ no ___

Scoring the Fast Burner Questionnaire

If you are a fast burner but suffer from kidney disease, osteoporosis or gout, the higher amounts of protein and purine rich proteins and vegetables (in the case of gout) are not recommended. In these cases, please follow your doctor's advice.

If you answered yes to eight or more questions, you are a classic *fast burner* type. The best way to approach a healthy diet is to follow these guidelines:

- A fast burner needs a diet that has a *higher fat and protein content* than slow burners. Remember that good fats are not the culprit in your diet when it comes either to being overweight or to developing heart disease: the artificial man-made fats are the problem, not the natural saturated fats in meats, when eaten in a balanced diet with the heart-smart monounsaturates and natural polyunsaturates.

- The fast burner can eat *protein with almost every meal,* but it should be of the heavier variety, such as beef, lamb, venison, or cold water fish like salmon. Dark meat fowl is also a good source of the heavier protein, and the fast burner also needs organ meats for their purine content.

- Always eat *meat with vegetables*—hearty vegetables like asparagus, cauliflower, spinach, mushrooms, beans, peas, and lentils are particularly suited for the fast burner.

- If you include potatoes or whole grains like rice in a meal, eat them with *butter* or *olive oil* to slow their release into your system. Like the slow burner, the fast burner must also keep in mind my warnings about excessive processed carbohydrate consumption. Eat vegetables and some whole grains with meals but *avoid processed carbohydrates* like bread, bagels, pasta, and crackers.

If you are a fast burner eating a low-fat, low-protein, or vegetarian diet, you may find that you are hungry all the time, and often are irritable or have mood swings. Protein, especially purine-rich protein foods like organ meats, in significant quantities is necessary for you to maintain a sense of equilibrium; it provides necessary nutrients and effectively reduces cravings for sweets. It also enters your bloodstream more slowly than carbohydrates, so it satisfies your hunger longer. Fats serve the important purpose of slowing down your overactive metabolism, as well as providing the essential fatty acids I spoke of earlier. Fats play another significant role in your diet if you are a fast burner: they literally help keep you warm. Fast burners tend to be very sensitive to cold weather, especially when there is not sufficient fat in the diet. Increasing dietary fat can help regulate your body's response to the cold!

If you scored five to seven yeses on the fast burner questionnaire, you tend toward being a fast burner and the dietary recommendations apply to you at least three to four days a week or at least two meals a day.

If you scored less than five yeses on either test, your metabolism level is balanced. If this is the case, you would do well to mix both lists of recommendations, varying your proteins between red meat and fowl and keeping your processed carbohydrate content low. Don't forget that blood type and ancestry will play a role in modifying your diet, so if you are a balanced type in between fast and slow, pay more attention to the blood type recommendations. Most importantly, you should be aware of how you're feeling; there will be times when you will want a heavier meal, and other times when a salad would feel just right. Don't ignore these messages you are getting from your body! If you feel like having a salad and you sit down to a meal of steak and potatoes, you won't feel very good at all afterwards. The same is true if you eat a salad and really feel like having meat and potatoes.

In Chapter 9, there are several lists of appropriate foods to eat and foods to avoid as well as an eating plan with a week's worth of sample menus, based on your individual body type. I've also included some general guidelines about eating the highest quality foods available, which apply equally to fast and slow burners. Keep in mind that your own body is still your best nutritional guide. You will need to pay attention to your own moods, feelings, and sensations when you eat different foods. If a food is on your list, but you find that it doesn't agree with you, feel free to eliminate it.

I have also provided a list of recommended vitamin and mineral supplements for the different types. Supplements are an important part of any diet; our hectic life-styles deplete our bodies of necessary nutrient stores and we can't depend on modern, chemically treated and processed foods to provide us with the kind of nutrients we need. As a balancing mechanism in both the fast and slow burner diets, vitamin and mineral supplements are an added necessity.

Ancestry As a Diet Modifier

Once you've determined whether you are a fast or slow burner, you can further personalize your ideal diet by taking into consideration your ancestral heritage. Most of us come from complicated backgrounds that mix several different nationalities. To make it easy, you may want to think of your ancestry in two very broad terms: **northern** and **southern**. People whose ancestry originated in the northern climates, like Scandinavia, northern and eastern Europe, and Canada, adapted to diets high in cold-water fish, red-meat animal protein, and root vegetables. Grains, tropical fruits, and vegetables were not the main components of their diets. The southern portion of the planet, however, produced a different range of foods: lighter-meat fish played a bigger role in the diet, as did light, water-based vegetables (lettuce, tomatoes, cucumbers, peppers), beans and legumes, and tropical fruits.

So, start to look at your family tree in terms of national origin to find clues about which foods might be best for you. For James and me, the Mediterranean diet (olive oil, pasta, beans), which has become so popular lowering cholesterol and heart disease, is not compatible with our northern and eastern European backgrounds. Consequently, neither of us have felt very good on a diet full of native Mediterranean foods, and now we know why. As I have said time and time again, we each carry a genetic blueprint of our nutritional needs, and a thorough examination of our own requirements will spell out the best ways to satisfy them. As you trace your national origin and all the different influences on your own nutritional requirements, you will continue to discover clues about the right foods for you.

Blood Type As a Diet Modifier

Another way to further individualize your diet is to make your food choices based on your blood type. Do keep in mind, though, the key principle of the fast and slow burner diets: Fast burners require a heavier diet that includes more protein and natural fats than do slow burners, who require a lighter diet including lean protein and greater amounts of carbohydrates than fast burners.

BLOOD TYPE O

Since blood type O's have the oldest blood type, they generally don't do as well with the new foods that were introduced in the human diet very late in our evolution. Therefore, both dairy foods and grains should be eaten sparingly by blood type O's. If you have a lactose intolerance, but you want to include dairy periodically in the diet for the sake of variety, you might want to select yogurt and other fermented dairy products like kefir, buttermilk, or acidophilus milk or use lactose-reduced dairy products. You can also purchase enzymes that will help you digest many products under the trade name Lactaid.

Instead of eating a lot of grains, fill your plate with more complex carbohydrate vegetables (including the fibrous, root, and starchy vegetables such as cauliflower, turnips, squash, and peas). Remember that O's also have a greater predisposition to celiac/sprue disease, which is the inability to digest gluten. If you do eat grains, try to stay away from the predominantly gluten-rich grains of wheat, rye, oats, and barley. Vary your grains to include buckwheat, quinoa, brown rice, and amaranth. Look for gluten-free breads, usually available at health food stores, made from rice, millet, or tapioca. Substitute whole-grain rice (all varieties except instant), millet, teff, quinoa, and amaranth for whole wheat. Spelt and kamut, ancient grains related to wheat, do contain gluten but may be better tolerated.

As the original hunter-gatherer blood type, blood type O has a higher need for protein than the other blood types, and therefore, the fast burner diet seems to be more ideal for blood type O than any other type. Protein sources should include organ meats and the richer red meats like beef, venison, and lamb, as well as poultry. Cold-water dark-meat fish is also good for blood type Os. If you are a slow burner and blood type O, stick to the leaner proteins listed for the slow burner: white meat poultry and the lighter fish. Whether fast or slow, blood type O's need a lot of protein, so try to eat meat, fish, or poultry at least twice a day. Fast burners can also handle a protein-rich breakfast.

The following is a list of foods that contain *gluten* and, therefore, should be avoided or limited by the blood type O's:

wheat, rye, oats, and barley
coffee substitutes made from grains like wheat, rye, oats, or barley
sauces made with wheat flour
packaged mixes made with wheat flour
luncheon meat, wieners, meatloaf, sausages, meat or fish patties
gravies made with wheat flour
canned and frozen foods thickened with flour, meal, or grains
cheese spreads containing cereal products as fillers
noodles, macaroni, pastas
commercial salad dressings made with wheat flour or other grains
oatmeal
rye, barley, and wheat breads; flour tortillas; biscuits
pastries, pies, commercial cakes, cookies
pancakes, waffles, toaster pastries
crackers made from wheat flour
cereal flour
soups thickened with wheat, flour, oats, barley, or rye and those containing barley
puddings, ice cream

BLOOD TYPE A

A's have a much lower need for protein in the diet than O's; however, that should be qualified by an understanding of the two A blood types, A-1 and A-2. People with blood type A-1 have lost the ability to make pepsin, a protein-digesting enzyme, in the digestive system, and they have compensated for this with an abundance of other enzymes that aid in the digestion of carbohydrates. A-1's are not well suited for a diet high in protein and full of meat and dairy products. Beans are also a bit of a problem for A-1's. Instead, their systems are better adapted to digest grains, but they should not overdo it. A wide variety of grains along with fruits, nuts, seeds, and eggs work well for the A-1's.

Blood type A-2's, on the other hand, have more of the necessary stomach acids and can handle more meats and seafoods in their diet. In general, A's are the only blood type suited to a vegetarian or near-vegetarian diet. Many of my clients who are blood type A prefer a vegetarian diet, although I warn them that such a diet often leads to an overdependence on grains, which can exaggerate a problem of gluten intolerance. Variety is the key to a healthy blood type A diet. If you are a blood type A and *not* particularly inclined to vegetarianism, you can eat the lighter proteins like chicken and turkey several times a week. The slow burner diet may be the best one for you to follow. Dairy products are also not part of the A's daily diet; keep them to a minimum or eliminate them completely. Like O's, A's may have a greater sensitivity to grain products as well, especially whole wheat. If you're a type A stick to rice, millet, buckwheat, kamut, spelt, and quinoa and gluten-free breads.

Blood type A's often suffer from digestive difficulties, primarily because of a lack of enough digestive enzymes. If this seems to be a problem for you, you may want to consider taking digestive enzyme or hydrochloric acid supplements. Type A's also should avoid lima beans since type A blood has a substance in it that causes the blood cells to agglutinate (clump) when lima beans are eaten. Clumped-together blood cells are harmful because they can cause circulatory problems and clot formation.

BLOOD TYPE B

Blood type B's share the diet of both the A and O, which means they can eat and happily digest a wide range of foods. Type B's can tolerate dairy products in moderation. Fermented dairy products like yogurt, kefir, and cottage cheese would be the best for type B's. Moderation is a key word for type B's, who can handle a little bit of everything but should not go overboard on any single type of food.

Blood type B's also have a particular element in the blood that causes it to agglutinate when certain foods are eaten. Chicken, buckwheat, sesame, and sunflower seeds all cause agglutination in type B blood and so should be avoided.

BLOOD TYPE AB

As the last-evolving blood type, AB is considered the modern blood type. AB's are very rare; they make up fewer than 4 percent of the American population. AB's fall somewhere in between A and B; in some cases they lean more toward the vegetarian A characteristics and in others toward the broader dietary range of the B. There should be significantly less emphasis on animal protein in the type AB diet, and most dairy foods can be tolerated in moderation.

Putting It All Together

So how will all this work for you? James and I, too, had to learn how to adapt our diets to adjust to these recommendations. I am a fast burner, and it is the ultimate irony that I was the nutrition director of a diet center focused on foods that are best suited for the slow burner. After much frustration, I have come to the conclusion that there is nothing inherently wrong with the Pritikin-type diets, which work for many people (some slow burners, particularly), but by learning what I now know about metabolic rates, I know that sort of light diet doesn't work for me.

Knowing that I'm a fast burner, I now make every effort to eat the foods recommended for a my type—the heavier proteins, healthy fats, more purine-rich vegetables, less processed carbohydrates. In addition, I'm a blood type B, which means I have a greater range of foods to choose from than the other blood types; I am also genetically more adapted to handle fermented dairy products. Because of my hectic schedule, I eat out often, but I have not had many problems finding the foods that agree with me. I try to eat sautéed liver once a week and, although I was hesitant at first (it's such an unpopular food, isn't it?), I find that I do feel more energetic when I eat it. Rather than order a vegetarian-style Caesar salad with sun-dried tomatoes, parmesan cheese, and a garlic- and cheese-based dressing, which had been my habit, I have started opting for the original Caesar salad. The anchovy- and egg-based salad is much more suited to my metabolic type and, although it meant breaking a habit, I've found the original Caesar is quite satisfying. I admit it's taken some time for me to retrain myself, but the results have been worth it. I have sardines two or three times a week for a quick but substantial lunch, and I no longer feel guilty indulging in a (hormone-free) hamburger. In addition, I've gotten off spices because I find I actually feel better when my food is simply prepared and spice-free.

My partner James, on the other hand, is a slow burner. He fared relatively well on the macrobiotic diet in the initial stages of healing his illness but, as a blood type O, had a much greater need for protein as a component of his maintenance diet. Now he makes sure he has fish three to four times a week, which is a protein he feels comfortable with after many years as a vegetarian. The fattier cold-water fish, like salmon and butterfish, although more strongly recommended for fast burners than slow, work well for James because as a blood type O he has a greater need for protein. In addition, those particular fish provide him with the important omega-3 essential fatty acids. As an American of English descent, James comes from a lineage that adapted to a diet high in cold-water fish, and, subsequently, high in omega-3.

The Continuing Quest

This is as good a place as any to tell you that I don't have all the answers. But the system I am suggesting is a good foundation that anyone can use to personalize his or her own dietary plan. It helps each of us begin to understand why our bodies need different foods to function at our best. Hopefully, with that understanding, we also will give ourselves permission to eat those whole foods our bodies have been craving. Even if the foods we crave are considered taboo by current dietary standards, I'm certain that our bodies have more wisdom about what's right for us than many of today's "experts."

Modern research is still fairly young in the area of biochemical individuality; we are all pioneers. I would love to see increased efforts in research about how best to individualize diet as well as health treatment in the years to come. Until then, use the guidelines in this chapter and keep listening to what your body is telling you to custom-design your diet.

Food for Thought

How quickly your body uses the food you eat is the most important determinant when choosing what kinds of foods are best for you. Would knowing whether you do better with heavier proteins like steak, ribs, and chops or lighter proteins like chicken and light fish help you stick to a simple, personalized diet when you go out to restaurants to eat?

You know best how you feel after eating certain foods. Think about the last time you ate a big plate of pasta with olive oil and vegetables. Did you feel uncomfortably full and yet hungry soon after? The last time you ate eggs, bacon, toast, and hash browns for breakfast, were you ready for lunch in a couple of hours or did it hold you until dinner time? Even if the fast and slow burner questionnaires give you trouble, you can just pay attention to how you feel—your energy level of hunger, and mood—after eating several typical meals. Once you know what to look for, you'll find out soon enough whether you are eating the right foods for you or not.

Your mother's Italian, your father's Irish. A Mediterranean-style diet, while occasionally satisfying, doesn't seem to be enough food for you when you have it on a steady basis. A consistent diet of meat and potatoes feels too heavy. What do you do? Balance. Mix. Pay attention to what your body is asking for. Note whether you are a fast burner (doing much better on the roasts and chops more often) or a slow burner (enjoying some light fish with a few vegetables and a salad). Some days a hearty meal will feel just right. On other days, a big salad with some cold chicken is just the ticket for you. Pay attention to how you feel!

You're a blood type O and need lots of protein in your diet. You've been a vegetarian so long you don't know where to start. First step: Visit the health food store for chemical-free, free range meats. If you're a fast burner, try the steaks and chops. If you're a slow burner, go for the chicken and turkey. Even though you think it might be difficult to incorporate meat into your diet, you'll find that after just a few meals, your body will be asking for more. If you can quiet the intellectual arguments going on in your head about the rightness of eating meat long enough to pay attention to how your body feels, you might find that your body knows better.

7

The Importance of Exercise

Now you have a better idea of your own individual blueprint for eating the right foods. You've looked at the rate of your own metabolism and blood type as well as ancestral background for clues about the foods best suited for you. Knowing which foods work with your own individual body mechanics gives you a basic framework for an eating plan that will provide you with the nutrients you need. You also know which foods are best for you individually to avoid, helping you in your goal of maintaining a weight level you feel comfortable with.

But is weight control the only reason to determine an individual eating plan? To be sure, keeping the fat off and being happy with the size and shape of our bodies are of major importance to most of us. But what about health? The easy answer is that without a lot of extra weight to carry around, the body is healthier. Eating the foods best suited to our bodies based on our own metabolism rate, ancestry, and blood type is the first step in the right direction. The next step, of course, is exercise.

Keeping Exercise Uncomplicated

Physical fitness has become a major industry in this country over the last 15 years or so. Just from an economic standpoint, take a look at the range of athletic shoes, workout clothes, fitness clubs, and aerobics classes and accessories that are available. When you consider the individual cash outlay now supposedly required to get fit, it's no wonder we keep putting off exercising, even though we know by now we're supposed to do it.

Exercise has become a complex ritual, requiring not only the proper attire and well-equipped facility, but time enough to go to the gym, work out for at least 45 minutes to an hour, shower, dress, and return to work or home. With a day that can include commuting to a full-time (physically sedentary but mentally demanding) job, taking care of children, preparing meals, and attending to all the other necessities of everyday life in a busy society, it's easy to think there is no time for exercising. Few of us spend any time at all in the sunshine and fresh air; even walking has become something we do only out of necessity.

Unfortunately, not many health club facilities are actually set up for the people who need them most: the overweight, the perpetually sedentary, and those recovering from illness and injury. More often than not, aerobics classes, with their complex choreography and fast pacing, are geared for those who are already fit and active. Little room is made for participants to modify the steps to their own comfort level, let alone for people who by their very body types do not do well with sustained, fast-paced exercise.

If you haven't begun an exercise program because you are intimidated by facilities, expenses, and classes that seem out of your range, then I have good news for you. You do not need a fancy health spa and daily hour-long aerobics classes, expensive workout clothing, or shoes. All you need is to get back to basics.

Recent studies confirm that a minimum of 30 minutes per day of aerobic exercise (which only means movement that increases your heart rate, not a dance class) is sufficient to provide the wonderful benefits of exercise that everyone is talking about.

Exercise without dieting is much more effective than dieting without exercise. That's right. Even if you don't want to change your eating habits one iota, you'll start feeling better just by pumping more oxygen into your system. But you'll soon find out that supporting your exercise with the right foods will make a big difference in how much progress you make in reaching your desired weight and improving your health.

The Benefits of Exercise

Aerobic exercise (which raises the heart rate and uses the large muscle groups of the body) is the best way for anyone and everyone to burn body fat. Aerobics in the form of structured, choreographed classes is not the only way to get aerobic exercise, though. Jogging, brisk walking, rowing, cross-country skiing, and bicycling are all great forms of aerobic exercise.

There are plenty of benefits to regular aerobic exercise. Exercising regularly (three to five days a week) increases circulation, tones the cardiovascular system, and brings additional oxygen into the system, which supports the function of all parts of the body. It beneficially stimulates the neuroendocrine (glandular) system and the production of brain neurotransmitters (providing a clear head and quick mind). Exercise also improves appetite (increasing or decreasing it depending on which you need), promotes better digestion, and facilitates elimination, as well as enhances the metabolic rate in order to burn body fat (provided that capacity has not been circumvented by an overload of carbohydrates in the system). Regular exercise also can control insulin production, a primary factor in weight gain. It also helps to control blood sugar levels without the need for insulin, and can significantly increase your glucose tolerance level.

Exercise stimulates the lymphatic system, which is integral to the removal of toxins from the body. When practiced on a daily basis, moderate exercise helps to lower cholesterol and blood pressure and can help thwart heart disease. None of these benefits are out of your reach. In general, thirty minutes a day of moderate aerobic exercise can be as simple and enjoyable as a brisk walk once or twice around the block. All you need to invest in is a pair of sensible shoes. If you have easy access to a pool, swim a few laps. You don't have to be an Olympian; just keep moving and maintain a steady pace for any stroke you like. If you have a yard, spend some time working in it: there is nothing like getting your hands in the dirt to bring a sense of calm and balance into your life. Digging and planting, raking, trimming, cleaning, mowing, and maintaining can provide endless muscle stimulation as well as an environment to be proud of.

Different Strokes for Different Folks

Just as we each have an individual dietary plan that works well with our own body, there is also a proper level of exercise that is appropriate for each different type of person. This exercise concept has been popularized by fitness expert Joanie Greggains. Slow burners (who ironically seem to have the least amount of physical energy) do best with fast-paced exercise that stimulates their metabolic rate. Fast burners, by contrast, have systems that run so high they are constantly in jeopardy of burning themselves out. Much of what they run on is nervous energy, not healthy, fat- or starch-burning energy. If you're a fast burner, you want to engage in exercise that will tone your body and burn fat but that won't stress your already depleted glands. Yoga, t'ai chi, swimming and gentle water exercises, peaceful and meditative walks, gardening, or easy, undemanding bike rides might be the best forms of exercise for you. Slow burners, on the other hand, will feel the most benefits from running, cycling, aerobics classes, and other more strenuous activities.

Different blood types also require different forms of exercise. The AB blood type and the B blood type persons do much better with a relaxing form of exercise like yoga, stretching, or t'ai chi, according to Dr. James D'Adamo. Overexertion is counterproductive for these types and can lead to exhaustion, especially of the endocrine glands. Blood type A's, who tend to have a sensitive immune system easily disturbed by stress, should also consider the milder forms of exercise, all of which promote mental clarity and have a calming effect. If you're one of those people who tend to get stressed out easily, an easy bike ride around the neighborhood might be better for your body than entering a 20-mile bike race. Gardening, swimming, and even light weight training are also good exercise possibilities for those who tend to be more high-strung.

On the other hand, D'Adamo suggests that O blood types tend to do better with vigorous exercise, which wards off fatigue and depression for them. If you have blood type O, you are a great candidate for regular participation in sports, whether you choose a company volleyball league or pickup basketball games at the neighborhood park. Regularly scheduled aerobics classes, long-distance bike rides, running, and fast-paced racquet sports would also be good for you.

What if you are a slow burner (needing more strenuous activity) but an A, B or AB blood type, who do better with the less rigorous activities? Pace yourself. Pay attention to your level of energy and your level of exhaustion. You might want to focus more on yoga or stretching exercises for two or three days, and in between have one or two days a week where you work a little harder, perhaps at an aerobics or dance class.

Eating to Get the Most out of Exercise

We have been conditioned throughout the Fitness Revolution to believe that a diet high in carbohydrates is necessary to sustain physical activity, and athletes often promote the wonders of the high-carbohydrate diet when working out. We've already seen, in this book's chapter on carbohydrates, that this is not entirely true. Remember, protein will raise your metabolic rate and help you access body fat, whereas carbohydrates (especially processed carbohydrates) raise your insulin level, preventing you from getting anything at all from stored body fat.

But carbohydrates do serve a purpose in any well-rounded diet, and the same holds true when exercising. Instead of skewing your diet too heavily in favor of carbohydrates when working out, be aware of your body type and adjust the amount of protein you eat. In addition, keep in mind the glycemic index rating of foods, which lists foods based on how quickly insulin is released into the bloodstream after they are eaten. (A glycemic index of common foods is listed on pages 128 to 129.) Foods with **low-glycemic** index will enter the blood stream *slowly* and therefore provide *sustained energy* over a longer period of time more than those with a **high glycemic index** which provide *quick bursts of energy.* If you are a fast burner your metabolism runs at a bit faster pace. So, low-index foods work a little faster in your system and high-index foods should be avoided unless combined with a slowing protein or fat because they have the effect of pouring gasoline on a fire when introduced into your system.

Slow burners, on the other hand, benefit from the high-index foods because the slow burner's slow metabolism rate acts as somewhat of a blockade to the quick burst of energy produced by these foods. Low-index foods act even more slowly in the slow burner body. Low-index foods include apples, cherries, dates, fresh figs, grapefruit, peaches, pears, plums, skim milk, plain yogurt, and kidney beans. These foods can help the fast burner sustain energy and are best eaten before long workout periods.

High-index foods, which provide a burst of energy because of their quick conversion to glucose, include raisins, potatoes, corn, and processed carbohydrates like corn flakes, bagels, and bread. A slow burner will find these foods provide a quick lift in the later stages of intense exercise or in stop-and-go workouts like basketball, weight lifting, and working out. Rice, spaghetti, rye bread, grapes, oranges, yams, and baked beans are in the middle range of the glycemic index and can be substituted for the high-index foods and eaten after working out.

Another important factor in working out is timing. Aerobic exercise is best done first thing in the morning when your stores of carbohydrates are low and your body taps into its own fat stores for energy when metabolism increases. After about 20 minutes of exercise any time of the day, your body moves into the "fat-burning phase," but if you exercise first thing in the morning, this phase will start sooner because you don't have other energy sources to draw from.

Staying Active for Our Health

The main thing for all body types to remember is that the human body is designed for regular daily activity. Circumventing that leads to weight gain and sluggish internal mechanics, including weakened immune and cardiovascular systems, a loss of skeletal flexibility, and a lack of physical and respiratory endurance. You don't have to become a fitness junkie or spend all your time (and money) at the gym. Just remember to take a walk every day.

GLYCEMIC INDEX OF FOODS

RAPID INDUCERS OF INSULIN SECRETION

Puffed rice	133
Rice cakes	133
Puffed wheat	133
Maltose	110
Breakfast cereal	100+

100

Glucose	100
White bread	100
Whole wheat bread	100

90–99

Grape-Nuts	98
Potato (russet)	98
Parsnips	97
Carrots	92

80–89

Quick rolled oats	80–90
Oat bran	80–90
Instant mashed potatoes	80
Honey	87
White rice	82
Brown rice	82
Banana	82
Potatoes (white)	81
Corn	82

70–79

All-Bran	74
Kidney beans	71

MODERATE INDUCERS OF INSULIN SECRETION

60–69

Raisins	64
Spaghetti	60
Whole wheat spaghetti	60
Pinto beans	60
Macaroni	64
Beets	64

50–59

Peas (frozen)	51
Sucrose	59
Potato chips	51
Yams	51

40–49

Oranges	40
Navy beans	40
Peas (dried)	49
Grapes	45
Whole grain rye bread	42
Sponge cake	46
Oatmeal (regular)	49
Sweet potato	48
Orange juice	46

REDUCED INSULIN SECRETION

30–39

Apples	39
Black-eyed peas	33
Chick-peas	36
Pears	34
Ice cream	36
Milk (skim)	32
Milk (whole)	34
Yogurt	36
No-fat peach yogurt	39
No-fat apple yogurt	39
Fish sticks (breaded)	38
Tomato soup	38

20–29

Lentils	29
Fructose	20
Plums	25
Peaches	29
Grapefruit	26
Cherries	23

10–19

Soybeans	15
Peanuts	13

JUICE RATINGS

Low—Peach, plum, cherry, grapefruit

Moderate—pear, oranges, apple, grape

High—Banana

(List reprinted with permission from Bio-Foods, Inc., Santa Barbara, Calif.)

Food for Thought

How can you squeeze exercise into a busy schedule? Take the stairs instead of the elevator. If you have several errands close together, walk to them, don't drive. If your parking lot is secure, park farther away from the front door than usual and walk. On your lunch break, walk around the block. Walk, walk, walk.

Don't have the time, inclination, or money to join a health club? Use videos at home. I particularly like the Joanie Greggains tapes. Get a few, mix and match. You can even work out to a holiday tape with Christmas favorites! Keep in mind your energy level—*fast burners* and blood types A, AB, and B do best with slower-paced, less strenuous workouts; *slow burners* and blood type O's can go all out with physical activity.

Even if you find yourself not fitting into these general guidelines, remember that you're a unique individual. Listen to your body's signals, and start exercising at whatever level you can; then proceed at your own pace.

Do you know you have to exercise? Yes. But do you have to make a big deal out of exercising? No. Walking the dog counts, raking the yard counts, and even doing the housework counts (as long as it's something like vacuuming, sweeping, moving the furniture, or painting the bathroom). Just be sure to be active and personalize the activity you do in whatever way suits you best.

8

Living in the Nineties

Thoughout this book, I've talked about eating the right foods based on your own unique makeup as a way to control your weight. The consequences of eating foods that your body is not well suited for can lead to more than merely extra pounds, however. The body's chemistry relies on an intricate web of complementing factors to keep it healthy and strong. Without the proper nutritional support that matches our unique metabolic needs, the immune system and the ability to ward off infection and disease can be compromised. This chapter explains some of the specific immune system stresses that we need to beware of in this day and age.

How Stress Affects our Bodies

How many times have you said, "I'm stressed out!" to your friends, your family, yourself during the last month? Stress became a big issue in those go-go 1980s, and it hasn't gone away. It's amazing how just one word can sum up so many sources of pressure and tension: home, family, and relationships; job performance, corporate structures, and deadlines; drastic changes in our personal and national economic outlook; crime, violence, and security issues. All these factors conspire to create a sense that we've lost control and the feeling that there is never enough time to get everything done. Our nerves are ragged, our tempers short, and our need sometimes just to get away from it all can become overwhelming.

There is definitely a physical component to the presence of stress. In addition to burdening the heart, blood vessels, and immune system, stress also adversely affects our adrenal glands (which regulate the body's minerals as well as work with the thyroid gland to produce and maintain the body's energy levels). There are basically three stages the adrenal glands go through during times of stress and each affects the body's general state of health in different ways.

1. **The Alarm Reaction** is the body's preparation for stress: the adrenal glands begin to hyperfunction, producing extra amounts of hormones to respond to the stress alarm. This is one of the normal functions for which the adrenals were designed. When the stress is removed, the adrenals quiet down and return to their normal functioning.

2. **The Resistance Stage** occurs when stress continues over a long period of time. The adrenals begin to adapt by actually increasing their size and function. In order to do this, however, energy will be drawn from the body's reserves. Nutrients not supplied by the diet will be siphoned off from reserve areas. This resistance stage can continue for weeks, months, and even years, until the body weakens due to lack of reserves of both energy and nutrients.

3. **The Exhaustion Stage** happens when the body's

reserves of both energy and nutrients are exhausted. The body can take only so much abuse. The antistress often expressed as fatigue or chronic tiredness, is one of the most common complaints in our country.

Lest you think emotional stress is the only form of stress we subject our adrenal glands to, think again. Physical stress, including physical injury, overwork, and lack of sleep, affects the adrenals as well. Any chemical substance, whether from environmental pollutants or diets high in refined and overprocessed foods, must be detoxified by our bodies, and this, too, puts stress on the adrenal glands. In addition, job stress, lack of or excessive exercise, and the use of stimulants such as coffee, sugar, and "recreational" drugs all contribute to adrenal burnout. Our bodies react in the same manner no matter what produces the stress.

Early warning signs of adrenal insufficiency include chronic low blood pressure, fatigue, low stamina, sensitivity to cold, and addictions to either sweet or salty foods. Those who consider themselves "night people" often suffer from adrenal exhaustion or burnout. These folks are usually tired when they get up and spend the better part of the day spiking their tired adrenal glands with caffeine, nicotine, sugar, sodas, or excessive exercise. At the end of the day, their burned-out but artificially stimulated adrenals are giving them energy to go all night. This cycle is a red flag for adrenal problems.

Nutrition Against Stress

Our nutritional needs skyrocket at the onset of tension and remain higher than normal during periods of prolonged stress. In the final analysis, whether the stresses come from mental or physical sources, nutrition is the key to fighting them. We need to fortify our body with the extra reinforcement it needs so that our reserves are not depleted during stressful periods. Adequate protein is one of the key remedies for a stressed-out body, as are a number of vitamins and minerals that can support and enhance adrenal function during this time. One of Uni Key's most requested and reordered products is called the Uni Key Adrenal Formula, which is a product that is made up of vitamins, minerals, and adrenal glandular tissue and that contains all the elements the body needs when under stress. This product is my personal guardian angel.

Magnesium, calcium, zinc, potassium, sodium, and copper are all depleted from body tissues as a direct result of stress. Surprisingly, the very best food sources of naturally balanced minerals come from the sea. Sea vegetables, sold in capsules or in dried form in health-food stores, provide high amounts of magnesium, potassium, phosphorus, iodine, and other key trace minerals like manganese, chromium, selenium, and zinc. Their extraordinary nutrient content and their tasty versatility make them an ideal side dish or condiment.

Of course, there are more familiar foods that you can choose from. These mineral-packed foods include all of the richly colored fruits and vegetables: green vegetables such as broccoli, collards, kale, and mustard greens; the yellow-orange vegetables, such as squash, pumpkin, carrots, and sweet potatoes; and fruits such as bananas, strawberries, and cantaloupe. Legumes are rich in iron, and eggs and meat are good sources of manganese and zinc. A surprising number of my clients suffering from adrenal burnout report strong cravings for chocolate, a food that is a fairly rich source of both magnesium and copper, two of the essential minerals required for energy production in the adrenals. Obviously, because of chocolate's high sugar content, it is not a great choice for mineral supplementation, but the cravings for it may graphically show the body's search for nutrients that have been lost due to stress.

The B-complex vitamins, known as the antistress vitamins, are crucial to take during stressful times. Even a slight lack of vitamin B_2 can cause a degeneration of the adrenal glands. Pantothenic acid nourishes the adrenals and a deficiency of this important B vitamin can cause atrophy. Many adrenal hormones are manufactured from cholesterol and cannot be made without the aid of pantothenic acid. In addition to supplements, the best sources of B-complex vitamins are desiccated liver, brewer's yeast, legumes, blackstrap molasses, and whole grains. Keep in mind that brewer's yeast, molasses, and grain products can cause yeast overgrowth, which I'll be discussing shortly, and should be taken in moderation. Brewer's yeast is also high in phosphorus, a calcium-competing mineral, so no more than 2 tablespoons per day is recommended for any one.

Vitamin C, zinc, and manganese are also important for healthy adrenal glands. The need for vitamin C has been found to increase dramatically during times of stress, when our bodies need as much as two and one half times more than normal. Amounts as high as 3,000 milligrams of vitamin C daily are not excessive during times of chronic stress. The body is better able to utilize vitamin C if it is taken in smaller doses throughout the day rather than taking it all at once. Fruits and vegetables rich in vitamin C include citrus fruits, cantaloupe, green peppers, and broccoli; rose hip tea is also a good source.

Both manganese and zinc are involved in numerous enzyme systems necessary for the utilization of vitamin C and the B-complex vitamins. Deficiencies in these minerals are prevalent today due to soil exhaustion, overprocessed foods, and careless cooking habits. Good sources of manganese include bananas, bran, whole grain cereals, nuts, and egg yolks. Good sources of zinc (a nutrient particularly important for women because it helps all aspects of reproduction) include lean red meats, eggs, brewer's yeast, liver, seafood, sunflower seeds, and mushrooms.

An interesting factor about stress is that when you are eating the right foods for your body, providing it with all the calories, nutrients, and exercise it needs, you tend to be able to handle stress a lot better. A body that is already depleted from a diet of empty calories, junk food, or the wrong foods for your individual system as well as a lack of regular physical exertion is going to have a difficult time handling the added pressures of a demanding boss, energetic children, or an unhappy relationship. Taking care of your body is one thing you do have control over; once you feel strong and healthy, you find it a lot easier to recognize solutions in other stress-producing areas in your life. And don't forget the wide range of relaxation techniques that have recently been popularized: yoga, deep breathing exercises, meditation, and massage are just a few of the ways you can take a break from your hectic life to relax and regroup.

The Need for Vitamins and Mineral Supplements

Based on all my experience as a nutritionist, I believe supplemental vitamins and minerals are now a necessity, not a luxury. In addition to combatting stress, vitamins and minerals provide a range of beneficial supports for all aspects of human biology. More than 80 million Americans are now supplementing their diets with vitamins and minerals. In the chapter on specific diets for the different metabolic types, I have included a list of recommended vitamin and mineral supplements. However, there are some nutrients that everyone, regardless of metabolic type or blood type, can benefit from. Although we should try to obtain our vitamins and minerals from the foods we eat, this is becoming more and more difficult. The advent of "modern" agricultural methods has left us with a legacy of poor soil. As the quality of our soil has declined, so has the quality of our food. Minerals that were once abundant in our soil, and consequently in our food, have been depleted. Selenium (an antioxidant), zinc, magnesium, calcium, and other trace minerals once abundant in our soils are now found only in marginal amounts, if at all, in many parts of the country.

One particular group of nutrients everyone can use, especially as protection against the toxins in our environment, are **antioxidants**. These nutrients work to block the oxidizing process in the body, a process that otherwise causes the production of free radicals, which damage and age cells. As I have said, free radicals are caused by normal processes in the body as well as by environmental factors like radiation, tobacco, smoke, pesticides, food additives, and air and water pollution. Antioxidants include the well-known vitamin C, vitamin E, and beta carotene, but other substances are even more powerful. A product called the Uni Key Antioxidant Formula, which I recommend to my clients, contains the most powerful 5 antioxidant substances from the grape, green tea, and natural botanical juice extracts, among other ingredients. (It is available through Uni Key Health Systems, 1-800-888-4353).

Vitamin C has been suggested in dozens of studies as a protector against various types of cancer (throat, pancreas, stomach, lung, esophagus, and mouth) as well as an enhancer of immune system response and a heart disease fighter. It may reduce the risk of cataracts and lessen the severity of cold symptoms. I prefer a time-release, buffered vitamin C that seems to be tolerated by most individuals. Individuals with hemochromatosis or iron overload disease will NOT want to include high doses of vitamin C in supplemental form because vitamin C is known to enhance iron absorption.

Candida—*A Growing Health Problem*

Stress is not the worst thing confronting us these days. In my opinion, yeast overgrowth is one of the major health problems we now face. Although its significance has been adamantly denied by large portions of the medical profession, it is interesting to note that, within the last several years, many yeast-fighting suppositories once requiring a prescription are now available over the counter and are heavily advertised on television. It has been estimated that one in three Americans harbor an overgrowth of *Candida*. Its symptoms include allergies, throat infections, joint swelling, memory loss, and repeated vaginal or bladder infections. Gastrointestinal disturbances like indigestion, constipation, diarrhea, and bloating also are common symptoms of *Candida* overgrowth, as are itching skin and acne, burning and tearing eyes, recurring ear infections, and nasal congestion.

In addition to the depletion of friendly bacteria in the gut due to broad-spectrum antibiotic use, there are several other causes of candidiasis. Most weight-watching women don't realize it, but the more fat-free products they eat, the more sugar they are unknowingly ingesting. Too much sugar in any form, including fruit and *processed carbohydrates,* can cause a yeast overgrowth in the system, as can a diet high in gluten-containing grains and yeast-related foods such as breads, pasta, beer, soy sauce, tomato sauce, vinegar, and cheese.

Remember, when sugars are consumed, blood sugar (glucose) levels rise quickly and the body produces insulin to carry the glucose to the cells. When blood sugar is too high, the defending cells of the immune system become semiparalyzed. These repeated stresses on our immunity eventually break it down and an overabundance of yeast begins to grow. Yeast cells grow and multiply rapidly in *all* sugars, including natural sugars like honey, molasses, and barley malt. In addition, if carbohydrates are not fully absorbed during digestion, some of them remain in the intestine, once again providing a fertile environment for the development of yeast. It is interesting to note that in my practice, I have seen complaints about *Candida*-related symptoms rise along with the popularity of the high-carbohydrate diet.

Birth control pills, steroids, and other drugs also can cause overproduction of yeast due to their immunosuppressive side effects. Another cause of yeast overgrowth is a deficiency in essential fatty acids; now you see why I stress the importance of having the right fats in your diet. In fact, Japanese researchers have found that oleic acid *interferes* with the yeast conversion to fungus. This monounsaturated fatty acid is found especially in olive, high-oleic sunflower and safflower, and avocado oils, and to a lesser degree in almond, apricot kernel, canola, peanut, and sesame oils. Essential fatty acids also decrease the permeability of vital tissues and organs, preventing yeast from spreading into the bloodstream from its normal intestinal and/or vaginal environs. Extremely low fat diets can create an ideal environment for yeast growth. Once again, the experts' advice of a low-fat diet failed to take into account this disastrous side effect.

Overcoming Candida *Naturally*

If you are plagued with frequent yeast infections, you may want to take a daily yeast fighting supplement until your internal flora is back to its normal levels. A homeopathic formula called Aqua Flora is an excellent, noninvasive form of treatment that I recommend to my clients as well as the Genesis Douche created by Dr. Richard Breitbarth. Both Aqua Flora and the Genesis Douche (purified water, aloe vera, grapefruit extractives and tea tree oil) are available through Uni Key Health Systems. As I've mentioned before, candidiasis is caused or aggravated by the steady ingestion of processed carbohydrate products (breads, crackers, bagels, muffins) and sugars (candies, cakes, cookies, etc.), so I suggest eliminating these foods completely from your diet and then only slowly reintroducing them, if at all. Sugars also include fruits, fruit juice, molasses, maple syrup, and honey, so be sure to cut these sugar sources from your diet as well. If you are bothered by yeast-related problems, you should also avoid all fermented foods such as alcoholic beverages, including wine and beer. Some individuals do well when restricting their intake of vinegary foods (pickles, mustard, green olives, sauerkraut, horseradish) during their recovery from candidiasis. Other foods to avoid include condiments like chutney and soy sauce, pickled and smoked meats, mushrooms, cheese, and dried and candied fruits. In addition to supplementing with acidophilus, add garlic to your daily diet, in the form of garlic supplements or fresh cloves added to food. In a study reported in *Mycologia* in 1977, researchers concluded that garlic inhibits the growth of yeastlike fungi.

As in the case of other cleansing diets I've mentioned, like juicing and macrobiotics, keep in mind that the dietary recommendations I've just listed are for the specific purpose of overcoming candidiasis; they are temporary and therapeutic in nature. Once you've cleared the yeast overgrowth out of your system, then you can begin your individualized diet plan with confidence.

Parasites—More Common Than Once Thought

Although this is not a particularly appetizing subject, I feel it's important to discuss the prevalence of foodborne and waterborne intestinal parasites. I spend a good amount of time with clients suffering from these infections. According to Theodore Nash, M.D., of the National Institute of Allergy and Infectious Diseases' Laboratory of Parasitic Diseases, parasitic infections are a major cause of illness in the United States. In fact, parasites may be another underlying cause of many of the unexplainable illnesses we are seeing in the 1990s. Allergies, immune dysfunction, recurring "stomach flu," and chronic fatigue are just a few of the myriad symptoms caused by parasites and bacteria. In my book *Guess What Came to Dinner* (Avery, 1993), I discuss in depth the different kinds of parasites we all are vulnerable to, the ways they spread, and the startling health complications they cause.

As I state in that book, parasites are an insidious public health threat in the United States today. Insidious, because so very few people are talking about parasites and even fewer people are listening. Insidious, because of the common misconception, among physicians and the general public alike, that parasites occur only in tropical Third World countries and areas traditionally associated with malnutrition and poor hygienic practices. Insidious, because physicians do not suspect, and therefore do not recognize, classic symptoms, and insidious, because even if physicians are aware of the threat, most use outdated and inadequate testing procedures, which result in underdiagnosis.

Several seemingly unrelated factors unique to the late twentieth century have contributed to the silent epidemic of parasitic contamination. Parasitic infections exist at a rate as high as 30 percent in day-care workers nationwide, due to diaper-changing practices and children who have direct contact with infected feces. Unsanitary conditions in Third World countries do indeed breed bacteria and parasites, and immigrants from those countries often bring along their uninvited internal guests, unwittingly spreading them when they take jobs in restaurant kitchens and child care facilities. Travelers abroad commonly find themselves with the unwanted souvenir of intestinal distress, and armed forces stationed overseas in the last several decades have brought several parasite-induced diseases back to our shores. Pets are also hosts to numerous parasites; in fact, there are 240 infectious diseases transmitted to humans by animals.

Another source of parasites and bacteria is the exotic foods that have become popular in the last few years. Ceviche, sushi, sashimi, Dutch herring, and steak tartare are all prepared raw or undercooked, posing a significant parasite risk. Any fish or animal meat that has not been sufficiently cooked can be a transmitter of a parasite or bacteria; 1993 saw a severe outbreak of *E. coli* bacteria in undercooked hamburgers in a fast-food outlet in Washington state, in which hundreds of people fell ill and some died.

Contaminated drinking water supplies are the most surprising cause of widespread infection in this country. *Giardia,* which has an affinity for *Candida,* is considered one of the most common waterborne parasites. Once seen mainly in international travelers drinking from contaminated water supplies and in campers and backpackers sipping from "pristine mountain streams" that were in reality contaminated by infected forest animals or raw sewage, *Giardia* has made its way across the country from the mountainous western regions to the East Coast. Unlike bacteria, *Giardia* is not killed by chlorine. Urban municipal water systems as well as those in rural areas can become contaminated through infected human sewage.

The municipal water system in the city of Milwaukee, Wisconsin, was threatened with contamination by the parasite *Cryptosporidium* in early 1993, causing at least a six-day water boiling advisory. Stomach cramps and diarrhea afflicted thousands of people there for up to two weeks. During the Great Flood of 1993, several municipal water systems in the Midwest were shut down due to malfunctions and the threat of possible bacterial and parasitic contamination. Washington, D.C., had its water supply shut off later that year due to cloudy water conditions, and several other cities throughout the country have had periodic water contamination problems. Also in 1993, researchers tested drinking water supplies in 14 states and found that one in four was contaminated with *Cryptosporidium.*

Parasitic infection is one of the most underdiagnosed health conditions I see in my clients. Symptoms vary depending on which of the hundreds of parasites or bacteria are present, but some of the more common ailments caused by these unwanted guests are constipation, diarrhea, gas and bloating, irritable bowel syndrome, joint and muscle aches and pains, anemia, allergic reactions, skin conditions, granulomas (tumorlike masses that encase destroyed larva or parasitic eggs), nervousness, sleep disturbances, teeth grinding, chronic fatigue, and immune dysfunction.

Parasites destroy cells in the body faster than they can be regenerated. They produce toxic substances that are harmful to the body and irritate or inflame body tissues, including the skin and intestinal lining. They are not something you want to learn to live with. Obviously, not every case of ill health can be blamed on parasites, but persistent, recurring symptoms that do not respond when treated for some other diagnosed ailment could be due to parasitic infection.

If you have trouble locating a specialist to help you, you can call Uni Key Health Systems to order a test kit that has been made available to my readers through an association between my office, Uni Key and a certified parasite laboratory. Some parasites can be eradicated only with harsh medications but others, including *Giardia,* respond to gentler natural formulas made of herbs following a careful intestinal cleansing program. You may choose to show the results to your health care practitioner (who hopefully has had experience with parasites) or choose to follow a natural program successfully used by many clients for several years.

Protecting Yourself from Parasites

It is possible to protect yourself from parasitic and bacterial infection. Don't drink untreated water. If you have well water or your municipal water system is small, located in a rural area, or close to contaminated ground water, buy bottled water. Don't eat uncooked or undercooked meat and fish. Practice preventive hygiene: wash your hands thoroughly and often, especially when handling raw food, pets, or diapers and when using the bathroom.

The manufacturers of Clorox bleach recommend the following procedure for cleansing kitchen utensils, cutting boards, knives, countertops, and sinks in order to kill *Salmonella* and other germs: Mix one sink full of water plus ⅛ cup regular Clorox liquid bleach. Wash the items, then soak them for two minutes in the Clorox solution. Rinse well and air dry. In addition, you can also soak out bacteria as well as chemical residues from vegetables, fruits, and cuts of chicken and beef with the following solution: one half teaspoon of Clorox to a gallon of water. Soak the foods in this solution for 15 to 20 minutes (30 minutes for thick-skinned fruits and root vegetables), then transfer to a second bath of fresh, filtered water and soak for another 10 minutes. Dry all foods thoroughly and store. The U.S. State Department has recommended such a formula for military families stationed in Turkey, China, and Southeast Asia to combat bacteria, parasites, and heavy metals. But such problems are by no means limited to countries overseas and Third World countries; America has many of the same problems and the same steps can be taken here to avoid them.

Overcoming Parasites Naturally

If you suspect you are infected with an intestinal parasite, there are several dietary measures you can take to make your internal environment less accommodating to these unwanted guests. An intestinal cleansing program is a good start; natural substances like psyllium husks, agar-agar, flax seeds, comfrey root, alginate, beet root, bentonite clay, citrus pectin, and papaya extract all act like a broom to sweep out the debris found in the digestive tract. Psyllium husks, flax seeds, and agar-agar are bulking agents that provide a rich source of water-soluble fiber that is without equal in removing accumulated wastes gently and effectively. Comfrey and beet root have a gentle laxative effect, and the enzymes in papaya extract help loosen the layers of mucus on the colon wall so that they can be eliminated.

Successful intestinal cleansing products you can find in most health food stores include Nature's Way Fibercleanse, Sonne's No. 7 and No. 9, Colon 8 by Ion Labs, Yerba Prima Internal Cleansing

Program, and Nature's Secret. Professionally administered colonic irrigation and home enemas can also be helpful in cleansing the colon.

The next step is to modify the diet to make the intestines inhospitable to parasites. A diet high in simple carbohydrates like sugar, white flour, and processed foods can provide the ideal feeding ground for bacteria and worms. Even so-called "natural" sweets—honey, barley malt, and fruit juice sweeteners and concentrates—taken in excess can provide instant food for parasites. Fiber-deficient foods initially may have provided a breeding ground for parasites, because they require more time to pass through the alimentary system. A sluggish transit time allows more food to decay and putrefy, thus producing stagnation in the colon and an inviting environment for parasites.

In my 20 years of experience with clients, I have found that a diet composed of 25 percent fat, 25 percent protein, and 50 percent *complex* carbohydrates (whole grains, starchy vegetables) works well if one is trying to cleanse a parasite-ridden body. The diet must have sufficient unprocessed oils (at least 1 to 2 tablespoons daily) from 100 percent expeller pressed safflower, sesame, flax, and canola oils. These oils lubricate the gastrointestinal tract and serve as a carrier for fat-soluble vitamin A, which best increases resistance to tissue penetration by parasite larvae. Foods rich in vitamin A such as cooked carrots, squash, sweet potatoes, yams, and greens should, therefore, be amply included in the diet.

Eating sufficient, properly cooked protein (meat, fish, chicken, eggs) is vital to a supportive therapeutic diet. And you will also want to restrict your intake of nuts, seeds, and legumes. These high-fiber foods, in the presence of parasitic infections, cause flatulence and irritate the gastrointestinal tract, which further prevents the absorption of nutrients. A high-fiber diet does help giardiasis, however; a water-soluble fiber supplement that is gentler to the gastrointestinal tract would be recommended instead. (Psyllium seed husks, rice bran, and oat bran are good substitutes.)

As you may have noticed in my discussion of how stress affects our adrenal glands, the popular low-fat, high-carbohydrate diet so revered in our culture often does not nourish the body enough to help it handle stress adequately. It also is the very diet that both *Candida* and parasites thrive on. A high-fiber diet is not the diet of choice when inflamed intestines and painful bloating are present as the result of either parasites or yeast infection.

Food for Thought

If "stressed-out" is the way you routinely answer the question, "How are you?" it's time to think about supporting your adrenal glands with vitamins, minerals, and the proper nutrients found in a healthy diet. Your body is responding to outside influences, but helping nourish your body on the inside is one of the most effective ways to help deal with those outside sources of stress and aggravation.

•

Do you have to quit your job, leave your partner, or move to a tropical island just to have a little peace and quiet? No. But you do have to eat foods and take vitamins and minerals that will support your stress glands. Will all your problems with the outside world go away? No, but they'll be a lot easier to deal with. And so will you, if you are always frying your nerve endings by the end of the day.

•

If you keep a stash of yeast-fighting suppositories in the medicine cabinet just so you'll be prepared for your next bout with *Candida*, have you asked yourself why this is happening to you so frequently? Is there anything you could be doing to prevent or overcome these problems? You bet. Chronic yeast infections can be controlled through diet, and the first thing to do is to avoid all forms of instant sugar. That means eliminating all those refined bread products (pasta, toast, muffins, bagels, and crackers), sugary desserts, fruit juices, and, yes, even those fruit-juice sweetened, fat-free cookies.

●

Are you constantly bothered by digestive discomfort? Parasites are a major health problem in this country these days. If you've tried every other way to combat bloating and gastrointestinal troubles, it's worth talking to your doctor about parasitic infection. And beef up on your hygiene habits: keep your house, especially the kitchen and bathroom, clean. Cities are especially dirty. Wash your hands before you eat no matter where you are.

9

What to Eat

Regardless of your blood type, ancestry, or metabolic rate, the following foods are not helpful to your body. They promote illness, they deplete your immune system and energy stores, and they can make you fat. They are unnatural foods and have no place in the human body.

No-No Foods for Both Slow and Fast Burners

General guidelines: EVERYBODY SHOULD AVOID THE FOLLOWING FOODS!

Trans or damaged fats: Eliminate margarine, shortening, and baked goods containing hydrogenated oils (such as commercially baked breads, cookies, cakes, and taco shells); commercial vegetable oils (soybean oil, corn oil); commercial mayonnaise and peanut butter; and all fried foods (especially french fried potatoes).

Oxidized cholesterol: Stay away from all smoked, dried, and aged meats and fish including bacon and ham; dried milk, dried eggs, and dried custard mixes; and aged cheese.

White refined sugar: Avoid cakes, cookies, candies, pies, and soft drinks. Also be careful of hidden sugars that are found in many processed foods like ketchup, canned soup, and toothpaste.

Sugar substitutes: Don't ingest aspartame (trade names are NutraSweet and Equal) and saccharin (Sweet'n Low). These are found in diet sodas, sugar-free yogurt, and diet cookies and candies, and are added to coffee.

Processed carbohydrates: Avoid all white flour products. Remember that processed carbohydrates (bread, crackers, bagels, pasta, muffins, etc.) act like simple carbohydrates in the body and should therefore be kept to a bare minimum in anyone's diet. Avoid building meals in which complex carbohydrates predominate; they should be in balanced amounts with protein foods and vegetables.

In addition, gluten-sensitive individuals (prevalent in blood type O's) should avoid wheat, rye, oats, and barley and substitute brown rice, millet, buckwheat groats, quinoa, and amaranth. Spelt and kamut, ancient grains, can often be better tolerated by those who are sensitive to wheat. However, they both contain gluten.

Beverages: Eliminate soda pop (diet, regular, and no-caffeine), powdered milk, and diet drinks and shakes. Don't drink coffee in excess of one to two cups a day or fruit juice in excess of one glass a day unless very physically active. Also avoid alcohol in excess.

Never drink untreated water from streams or lakes, no matter how pristine you think they are. Spring water, well water, and all ground water sources are possible carriers of *Giardia,* an intestinal parasite prevalent in this country as well as in Russia, Europe, Asia, and South America. Get a good home water filter system that blocks microorganism cysts like *Giardia* and *Cryptosporidium* if your home water system is fed from a well or spring. Use a portable water filter when camping or backpacking or bring bottled water.

Protein: Avoid all raw eggs and raw meat and fish dishes, such as steak tartare, ceviche, and sushi. Also avoid all rare-cooked meats and fish. Raw flesh foods can contain numerous bacteria (such as *Salmonella* and *E. coli*) and parasites (such as tapeworms). Only thorough cooking at a sufficiently high heat (180 degrees Fahrenheit, minimum) can kill these organisms. Farm-raised salmon, shrimp, and rainbow trout may have had less exposure to marine pollutants but also have a lowered amount of essential fatty acids than their naturally harvested counterparts. Refer to the instructions for the special food cleansing bath in the last chapter for cleaning naturally harvested fish.

Vegetables: Avoid canned vegetables.

Seasonings: Avoid all irradiated herbs and spices. Avoid commercial salt because it is chemically cleaned and has added aluminum silicate to prevent caking and dextrose (a sugar) to cover up the bitter taste of the aluminum. (Use sea salt instead).

User-Friendly Cookware Tips

Sometimes, even your pots and pans can add unwanted ingredients to your food. So if you are using a microwave, make sure to use only containers labeled "Safe for Microwaving." Certain plastic containers, such as margarine tubs, for example, can melt and actually be absorbed into your food. But you shouldn't be using margarine anyway, after reading the section on detrimental trans fats, remember?

Avoid cooking highly acidic foods in aluminum pans. Foods such as sauerkraut, rhubarb, and tomato sauce can oxidize aluminum and absorb it. Excessive aluminum in the body (which comes mainly from aluminum hydroxides in antacids) can affect the body's utilization of calcium and phosphorus and has been associated with Alzheimer's disease. Unlined copper pots and pans should also be avoided. Although copper is a great heat conductor, unlined copper can leach into food, affecting vitamin C utilization in the body and causing nausea and vomiting.

The most desirable cooking utensils are made of high-quality stainless steel, Corning Ware, Pyrex, and tinted glass. Cast iron is also acceptable unless you are an individual with hemochromatosis (iron overload in the body), as cooking in iron pots and pans can add a significant amount of iron to the food. (This is especially true if the food is acidic, like apples or tomatoes.) Even certain stainless steel cookware can leach iron (as well as nickel and chromium) into food when exposed to acid-based foods.

James and I personally use and recommend Royal Prestige cookware, because of the unique seven-layer construction that prevents any metal at all from leaching into the food. Royal Prestige's minimum moisture method allows food to cook without nutrient-depleting water or excessive fat. The special vacuum sealing allows food to cook at 180 degrees—the temperature that destroys bacteria, germs, and parasites. (Call Uni Key at 1-800-888-4353 for more information.)

Slow Burner Food Formula

Now you are ready to put all the dietary concepts of *Personalized Health* together in an easy-to-follow daily plan. Here is the **daily slow burner prescription** that will insure optimum nutrition for the slower metabolic type:

- 2 tablespoons of essential and healthy fats
- 4 to 6 ounces low-fat, low-purine protein
- 4 or more servings of vegetables
- 2 to 4 servings of fruit
- 4 or more portions of complex carbohydrates
- 2 nonfat dairy servings (optional, if tolerated)

SLOW BURNER FOOD CHOICES

The *Slow Burner* Food Choices Lists for essential fats, proteins, vegetables, fruits, complex carbohydrates, and dairy products will help to illustrate the right foods for this metabolic type and also teach you balanced portions for each serving of food.

Essential and Healthy Fats: A combined total of *two tablespoons* can be chosen among the following recommended fat choices. Flax, safflower, sunflower, sesame, and corn oils are best used in the unheated form (with salads, for example). Flax oil is absolutely delicious drizzled on air-popped popcorn and brown rice. You can also use it to jazz up baked potatoes, because it tastes like drawn butter. Although the menu plans do not mention flax oil particularly, feel free to use it any time a healthy oil is called for, in its uncooked form. Use canola, peanut, or olive oil for cooking. Spectrum Spread, made with canola oil, is one of a growing number of healthy spreads on the market that do not contain the dangerous trans fats so prevalent in margarine and vegetable shortenings. Use it with confidence on toast and steamed vegetables. Remember to choose expeller-pressed oils rather than commercially processed; certified organic is best.

Feel free to mix and match the following essential and healthy fats. I've listed each source for its equivalent to 1 teaspoon, unless the source has a different measurement that is otherwise noted. Combine them in any way you like to achieve 2 tablespoons.

NATURAL OILS

Flax

Safflower

Sunflower

Sesame

Corn

Peanut

Canola

Olive

MAYONNAISE (safflower- or canola-based)

NUTS AND SEEDS (dry-roasted or home-toasted)

Cashew	4 nuts or 1 tablespoon
Peanut	20 small or 10 large
Pistachio	15 nuts
Pumpkin	1 tablespoon
Sesame	1 tablespoon
Sunflower	1 tablespoon

Proteins: Include a total of *4 to 6 ounces daily* from any combination of the following protein choices. They are listed in equivalents of 1 ounce, so you can mix and match any way you like your total daily intake. Again, those with no amount listed are equivalent to one ounce. (Remember, these are not portion sizes. The measurements listed equal 1 ounce and are provided to make it easy for you to combine different foods.) It's best to spread out protein foods throughout the day, eating some at every meal. Try to use free-range and hormone-free meats and poultry whenever possible, as well as fertile eggs from free-range chickens. These meats and eggs have as much as five times the amount of essential fatty acids (EFAs) and a greatly reduced amount of hard cholesterol fat than their caged and feed-lot counterparts. There are several companies that offer organically raised poultry. These include Shelton Farms, Harmony Farms, Foster Farms, and Youngs Farm. One of the most widely available suppliers of organic beef is Coleman Natural Beef, based in Denver, Colorado.

NONFAT CHEESE

Dry curd, skim, 1% or less cottage cheese	¼ cup
Lifetime Swiss, mozzarella, mild cheddar, Monterey Jack	1 ounce
Grated Parmesan	2 tablespoons

EGGS

Whole	1 egg
Whites	3 whites

FISH AND SEAFOOD

   Cod

   Sole

   Flounder

   Scrod

   Haddock

   Turbot

   Perch

   Canned tuna (solid white albacore)   ¼ cup

POULTRY

   White meat turkey

   White meat chicken

   Cornish hen (without skin)

LEAN BEEF

   Round, sirloin, flank steak

   Tenderloin

   Chipped beef

LEAN VEAL

   Chops and roasts

OTHER

   Tofu (2½ × 2¾ inches)

Vegetables: Include a daily total of *4 or more servings* from the list below. One serving should be ½ cup cooked or 1 cup raw unless otherwise indicated. Fresh salads should be eaten every day and veggies like cucumbers, tomatoes, and sprouts can be used for snacks. Since high amount of potassium can help the *slow burner* metabolism to speed up, potassium-rich vegetables like Jerusalem artichokes, squash, and tomatoes should be highlighted.

   Bamboo shoots

   Beans (green, wax, Italian)

   Beet

Broccoli

Brussels sprouts

Cabbage

Eggplant

Greens (lettuce, collard, mustard, turnip)

Jerusalem artichokes (sunchoke)

Jicama

Kohlrabi

Onions

Parsley

Peppers

Radishes

Rutabaga

Snow peas

Sprouts (alfalfa, radish, mung, clover)

Squash (yellow or crookneck, Italian or
  zucchini, spaghetti, chayote)

Tomatoes

Vegetable juice	½ cup
Watercress	
Water chestnuts	6 whole

Fruits: These fruits are also recommended snacks to be enjoyed between meals. *Two to four servings a day* are recommended, and remember to include citrus fruits and bananas frequently because of their high potassium level. Measurements listed are one serving size. Avoid frozen or canned fruits, especially those with additives, chemical preservatives, and sweeteners. Certified organic fruits are best if you can find them.

Apple	1 small
Apple butter (sugar-free)	2 tablespoons
Apple juice or cider	⅓ cup
Applesauce (unsweetened)	½ cup

Apricots (fresh)	2 medium
Apricots (dried)	4 halves
Banana	½ small
Berries (boysenberry, blackberry, blueberry, raspberry, strawberry)	¾ cup
Cantaloupe	⅓ melon
Cherries (large raw)	12
Dates	2
Figs (raw)	2
Figs (dried)	1½
Fruit cocktail (in own juice)	½ cup
Fruit preserves and spreads (sugar-free)	2 tablespoons
Grapefruit	½
Grapefruit juice	½ cup
Grapes (small)	15

Complex Carbohydrates: Include *four or more servings* from the following varieties on a daily basis. You can add or subtract servings depending upon your ability to metabolize carbohydrates as well as on how physically active you are. Measurements listed are serving sizes. Cereals and other foods made from gluten-based grains (wheat, rye, oats, and barley) should be kept to a minimum and rotated with other nongluten grains. Also, emphasize the starchy vegetable group of foods.

STARCHY VEGETABLES

Chestnuts (roasted)	4 large or 6 small
Corn (on the cob)	1 (4 inches long)
Corn (cooked)	⅓ cup
Lima beans (fresh)	½ cup
Parsnips	1 small
Peas (frozen)	¾ cup
Potatoes sweet (yam)	⅓ cup
Potatoes, white (baked, boiled)	1 small

Potatoes, white (mashed)	½ cup
Pumpkin	¾ cup
Squash (winter, acorn, butternut, buttercup)	1
Succotash	½ cup

BREADS

Bagel (whole wheat, spelt)	½ small
Bread, rye, pumpernickel, whole wheat	1 slice
Breadsticks, whole grain	4 (7 inches long)
Bun, hamburger or hot dog, wholegrain	½
Croutons, whole grain	½ cup
English muffin, whole grain	½
Pancakes, whole grain	2 (3-inch diameter)
Pita bread, whole grain	½ (6-inch pocket)
Rich cakes, whole grain	2
Roll, wholegrain	1 (2-inch diameter)

CEREALS AND GRAINS

Barley (cooked)	½ cup
Bran flakes	½ cup
Bran (unprocessed rice or wheat)	⅓ cup
Buckwheat groats (kasha, cooked)	⅓ cup
Cornmeal (cooked)	½ cup
Couscous	⅓ cup
Cream of rice (cooked)	½ cup
Grape-Nuts	¼ cup
Grits (cooked)	½ cup
Millet (cooked)	½ cup
Oatmeal	½ cup
Popcorn	3 cups
Puffed rice, wheat, millet, or oats	1½ cups
Rice (brown, cooked)	⅓ cup

Rice (wild, cooked)   ½ cup

Shredded wheat biscuit   1 large

Tapioca   2 tablespoons

CRACKERS

Matzoh, whole wheat   ½ 6 × 4 inches)

Pretzels, whole grain   1 large

Rice wafers, brown rice (Westbrae)   4

Rye crisp bread crackers (Wasa)   2

Wheat crackers, whole wheat (Ak-Mak)   4

FLOURS

Arrowroot

Buckwheat

Cornmeal

Cornstarch

Potato

Rice

Soya powder

Whole wheat

LEGUMES

Beans, dried (cooked) lima, navy,
    pinto, kidney, black   ⅓ cup

Beans, baked, plain   ⅓ cup

Lentils, dried (cooked)   ⅓ cup

Peas, dried (cooked)   ⅓ cup

Peas, fresh (cooked)   ½ cup

PASTA

Noodles, macaroni, spaghetti (cooked)   ½ cup

Noodles, rice (cooked)   ½ cup

Noodles, whole-wheat (cooked)   ½ cup

Pasta, whole-wheat (cooked)   ½ cup

Dairy: If you are going to use dairy at all, do not exceed the suggested *two servings a day* from this group. Dairy products are excessively high in calcium, which will slow down the metabolism of the *slow burner* even more than it already is. If you have difficulty digesting milk (lactose intolerance is especially common among blacks, Native Americans, Mexicans, Asians, and Jews of Eastern European descent), then fermented dairy products like yogurt, kefir, buttermilk, and acidophilus milk may be more easily tolerated. You can also purchase enzymes under the trade name Lactaid to use in regular milk.

Milk: nonfat cow's milk, goat's milk,
   buttermilk, acidophilus milk   1 cup

Yogurt: nonfat cow's milk, plain; goat's
   milk, plain; kefir   1 cup

Seasonings: If you find the meal plans a little too bland for your taste buds, feel free to spice them up. *Slow burners* do particularly well with condiments such as curries, chiles, hot sauces, and cayenne pepper, but use a light hand in adding them to your food. A little goes a long way, metabolically speaking.

The Basic Slow Burner Eating Plan: A Week of Sample Menus

The following is a week-long menu plan to get you started eating for your metabolic type. Each menu incorporates the nutritional information outlined at the beginning of this chapter. Below are some notes about modifying the diet based on your blood type.

• If you have type O blood, you may feel better with a little lean protein at every breakfast. If you are lactose intolerant, eliminate the dairy component or try lactose-reduced dairy products that include the enzyme product Lact-aid that are now on the market. If you are gluten sensitive, use gluten-free breads made from rice, millet, and tapioca to replace whole-wheat breads, crackers, and pita. Spelt and kamut, although they contain some gluten, may be tolerated.

- Type A's can go for a more vegetarian version of the diet but should not eliminate animal protein completely.
- Type B's should substitute turkey or fish for chicken in the menus and can eat yogurt and fermented dairy products.
- Type AB's with more of an A food orientation should follow the A guidelines; those AB's who lean toward B characteristics can add the fermented dairy products to their diet.

MONDAY

BREAKFAST:

½ Grapefruit

Egg-white omelet with onions, parsley, and green peppers

2 slices sprouted whole grain toast with

1 teaspoon Spectrum Spread

1 cup coffee

LUNCH:

2 ounces grilled chicken breast

Ratatouille made with

1 teaspoon sesame oil

Steamed barley and rice

DINNER:

3 ounces fillet of sole

Medley of leeks, zucchini, and yellow squash

Mixed sprout salad with

1 tablespoon safflower/lemon dressing

TUESDAY

BREAKFAST:

¾ cup blueberries with
½ cup old-fashioned rolled oats and
4 ounces skim milk
1 cup coffee

LUNCH:

3 ounces tofu, water chestnuts, bok choy, broccoli, and red
  peppers, stir-sautéed in
1 tablespoon peanut oil
½ cup sauerkraut
½ cup buckwheat noodles

DINNER:

3-ounce turkey burger on
½ whole grain bun
½ cup mashed potatoes with
1 teaspoon Spectrum Spread
Grilled eggplant with sweet peppers and onions
Lettuce, cucumber, and radish salad with
1 tablespoon olive oil and lemon juice dressing

WEDNESDAY

BREAKFAST:

1 Orange
1 Poached egg
2 slices whole rye toast with
1 teaspoon Spectrum Spread
1 cup coffee

LUNCH:

3 ounces albacore tuna salad with

2 teaspoons canola mayonnaise, sweet relish, and onion powder

2 Rice cakes

Romaine lettuce with apple cider vinegar

DINNER:

2 ounces roast Cornish game hen

½ cup wild rice and leek stuffing

Warm red cabbage with caraway seeds and

1 tablespoon virgin olive oil and lemon juice dressing

THURSDAY

BREAKFAST:

½ Banana with

1 cup nonfat yogurt and

3 tablespoons toasted wheat germ

1 cup coffee

LUNCH:

3 ounces breast of turkey on

2 slices rye bread with

1 tablespoon safflower mayonnaise and

Sprouts, mustard, and onions

Sliced tomatoes

DINNER:

3 ounces baked scrod with piquant tomato sauce

1 Baked potato brushed with

1 tablespoon virgin olive oil

Green beans

Chopped lettuce, parsley, and scallions with

1 tablespoon sesame and vinegar dressing

FRIDAY

BREAKFAST:

1 Stewed apple with cinnamon and

2 tablespoons raisins

1 cup coffee

LUNCH:

Vegetable broth

2 ounces shredded seafood salad stuffed in tomato

4 Whole grain crackers

Leafy salad with

1 tablespoon peanut oil dressing

DINNER:

4 ounces broiled halibut

Braised brussels sprouts, pearl onions, and nutmeg topped with

1 tablespoon safflower and lemon dressing

1 cup sweet potato

SATURDAY

BREAKFAST:

½ Grapefruit

½ cup 7-Grain cereal

4 ounces nonfat milk

1 cup coffee

LUNCH:

Greek salad made with

2 ounces feta cheese, tomatoes, Bermuda onions, and parsley and

1 tablespoon olive oil and lemon dressing

2 Rice cakes

DINNER:

1 cup whole grain pasta and

4 ounces turkey meatballs with marinara sauce

Mixed greens with

1 tablespoon corn oil dressing

SUNDAY

BREAKFAST:

½ cup Kashi with

1 cup nonfat yogurt

1 cup coffee

LUNCH:

Gazpacho

Sliced Jerusalem artichokes

Egg salad made with 2 eggs, chopped celery, onions, and

1 tablespoon canola mayonnaise on

2 slices whole rye or spelt bread

DINNER:

3½ ounces chicken cutlet

Baby vegetable melange: 1 small potato, baby carrots, green
beans, zucchini

Endive and Bermuda onion salad with

1 tablespoon safflower/lemon dressing

- Beverages with meals include water, herbal tea (alfalfa is best for this type), Kukicha (Japanese twig tea), and coffee substitutes. One cup of coffee per day is okay for most slow burners.
- Drink at least eight glasses of pure water daily between meals. Herbal teas and coffee substitutes can be used as beverages but are not substitutes for water.
- Snacks: Choose snacks of mostly low-fat, light foods like veg-

gies, fruits, and complex carbohydrates (for examples, cucumber rounds, an orange, whole grain rye crackers, or, occasionally, a piece of part-skim mozzarella cheese).

Slow Burner Vitamin and Mineral Supplements

Remember, again, that this list is to be used as a basic foundation. Because each of us is unique and has different nutritional needs, please consult a qualified health practitioner to determine the right balance of vitamins and minerals for you.

Note: These vitamins and minerals are best taken with food once a day unless otherwise noted.

Vitamin B_1—50 mg
Vitamin B_2—50 mg
Niacin—100 mg
Vitamin B_6—50 mg
Para-aminobenzoic acid (PABA)—100 mg
Ascorbic acid—1,000 mg 3 times daily
Vitamin D—100 IU
Chelated potassium—99 mg 2 times daily
Chelated magnesium—200 mg 2 times daily
Chelated manganese—30 mg
Iron—18 mg

Fast Burner Food Formula

Here is the **daily fast burner prescription** that will insure optimum nutrition for the fast metabolic type:

- 3 tablespoons essential and healthy fats
- 6 to 8 ounces animal protein (include heavier, high-purine sources four times a week)
- 4 or more servings of vegetables

- 1 to 2 servings of fruit
- 2 or more servings of complex carbohydrates
- 2 full-fat servings of dairy (optional, if tolerated)

Essential and Healthy Fats: A combined total of *3 table-spoons a day* can be enjoyed from this group by the fast burner. Use olive oil for salads and both olive oil and butter for cooking. For high-heat stir-frying, choose the high-oleic safflower and sunflower oils. Expeller-pressed, organic oils are best. Certified raw, organic butter, cream, and cream cheese are desirable, if they are tolerated.

Feel free to mix and match the following essential and healthy fats. Unless otherwise noted, each source of fat on the list is measured as 1 teaspoon. Combine them in any way you like to achieve 3 tablespoons. (Keep in mind that the measurements listed are not portion sizes but the equivalent of 1 teaspoon.)

NATURAL OILS

Almond

Avocado

Canola

Olive

Sesame

Safflower (high-oleic)

Sunflower (high-oleic)

OTHER FATS

Avocado	½ small
Butter	
Bacon, Canadian	1 slice
Cream, light, sour	2 tablespoons
Cream, heavy, whipped	1 tablespoon
Coconut, shredded	2 tablespoons
Cream cheese	1 tablespoon
Olives	10 small or 5 large
Mayonnaise (canola-based)	

Proteins: Include a total of *6 to 8 ounces of protein daily* in any combination from the following list of protein choices. Remember that all animal protein sources are acceptable for the fast burner, but you should include those foods rich in purines at least four times a week for their high-energy properties. (Purine-rich foods are noted with an asterisk.) Try to use free-range and hormone-free meats and poultry and harvested fish whenever possible for the higher amounts of nutrients they provide compared to their commercial counterparts. Fast burners also may use nitrate-free and nitrite-free frankfurters (beef, chicken, turkey).

FISH AND SEAFOOD

Carp

Catfish

Mackerel

Salmon

Shark

Swordfish

Trout

Whitefish

*Caviar, fish roe
*Herring

*Oyster, clam, shrimp, mussels, scallops   5 small

*Anchovy, well rinsed   3 medium

Canned tuna, chunk light   ¼ cup

Lobster

*BEEF

Rib, chuck, rump roast

Cubed, porterhouse, T-bone steak

Prime rib

Liver, sweetbreads, heart, kidneys

Frankfurter   1

POULTRY

    Dark meat chicken

    Dark meat turkey

    Frankfurter, chicken, or turkey   1

*VEAL

    Cutlet

*LAMB

    Chops, leg, roast, patties

*WILD GAME

    Pheasant, goose, duck

    Venison

OTHER

Peanut Butter	1 tablespoon
Almond Butter	1 tablespoon

Vegetables: Include a daily total of *four or more servings* of vegetables. A serving is ½ cup cooked or 1 cup raw. Purine-rich vegetables (marked with an asterisk) and those higher in vitamin A and calcium are best for the fast burner. Sea vegetables are particularly high in calcium, and so are good choices for fast burners, who need calcium to help slow down their overactive metabolism.

    *Asparagus

    *Artichokes (globe or French)

    Artichoke hearts

    Broccoli

    Brussels sprouts

    Cabbage

    Collards

    Endive

    *Mushrooms

    Kale

Parsnips

Okra

Parsley

Rutabaga

Turnip greens

Squash

*Cauliflower

*Spinach

SEA VEGETABLES

Dulse

Hijiki

Kombu

Nori

Fruit: Fast burners should limit fruit to *one to two servings a day.* Fruit is best eaten with a protein or fat, such as nut butter, yogurt, or a slice of cheese. Citrus fruits in particular should be avoided by the fast burner because its high potassium level speeds up the metabolism.

Apricot, medium, raw	4
Cranberries, unsweetened	½ cup
Nectarine	1
Cherries	12
Peach	1
Blueberries	¾ cup
Cantaloupe	⅓ melon
Papaya	1 cup
Pear	1
Watermelon	1¼ cup

Complex carbohydrates: The fast burner can eat *two or more servings a day* of grains, cereals, and starchy vegetables. Amounts given are serving sizes. Remember to slow down the speedy effect of these foods by combining them with a fat, such as butter, nut butter, oil, or cheese. Also, try to purchase breads made from sprouted grains, because unsprouted grains contain phytates, which tend to lower calcium and increase oxidation (metabolism) rates. Your health food store should have many kinds of sprouted grain breads to choose from. The purine-rich carbohydrates, which you should try to eat several times a week, are noted with an asterisk.

STARCHY VEGETABLES

Chestnuts (roasted)	4 large or 6 small
Corn (on the cob)	1 (4 inches long)
Corn (cooked)	⅓ cup
Lima beans (fresh)	½ cup
Parsnips	1 small
Peas (fresh)	¾ cup
Potatoes (sweet, yam)	⅓ cup
Potatoes, white (baked, boiled)	1 small
Potatoes, white (mashed)	½ cup
Pumpkin	¾ cup
Squash (winter: acorn, butternut, buttercup)	1
Succotash	½ cup

BREADS (sprouted grain)

Bagel, whole wheat, spelt	½ small
Bread, rye, pumpernickel, whole wheat	1 slice
Breadsticks, whole grain	4 (7 inches long)
Bun, hamburger or hot dog, whole grain	½
Croutons, whole grain	½ cup
English muffin, whole grain	½
Pancakes, whole grain	2 (3-inch diameter)
Pita bread, whole grain	½ (6-inch pocket)
Rice cakes, whole grain	2
Roll, whole grain	1 (2-inch diameter)

CEREALS AND GRAINS

Barley (cooked)	½ cup
Bran flakes	½ cup
Bran (unprocessed rice or wheat)	⅓ cup
Buckwheat groats (kasha), cooked	⅓ cup
Cornmeal (cooked)	½ cup
Couscous	⅓ cup
Cream of Rice (cooked)	½ cup
Grape-Nuts	¼ cup
Grits (cooked)	½ cup
Millet (cooked)	½ cup
Oatmeal	½ cup
Popcorn	3 cups
Puffed rice, wheat, millet, or oats	1½ cups
Rice (brown), cooked	⅓ cup
Rice (wild), cooked	½ cup
Shredded wheat biscuit	1 large

CRACKERS

Matzoh, whole wheat	½ (6 × 4 inches)
Pretzels, whole grain	1 large
Rice wafers, brown rice (Westbrae)	4
Rye crisp bread crackers (Wasa)	2
Wheat crackers, whole wheat (Ak-Mak)	4

FLOURS

Arrowroot
Buckwheat
Cornmeal
Cornstarch
Potato
Rice
Soya powder
Whole wheat

*LEGUMES

Beans, dried (cooked) lima, navy, pinto, kidney, black	⅓ cup
Beans, baked, plain	⅓ cup
Lentils, dried (cooked)	⅓ cup
Peas, dried (cooked)	⅓ cup
Peas, fresh (cooked)	½ cup

PASTA

Noodles, macaroni, spaghetti (cooked)	½ cup
Noodles, rice (cooked)	½ cup
Noodles, whole wheat (cooked)	½ cup
Pasta, whole wheat (cooked)	½ cup

Dairy: If you are not lactose intolerant or allergic to milk, *two or more servings* of dairy products should be included in your daily diet. Remember to choose the full-fat version, not skim or low-fat. The fat content is actually what is most beneficial to the fast burner because of its slowing effect. The high calcium content of dairy foods also is good for the fast burner for the same reason: it slows down the metabolism. Be sure to look for the highest quality dairy products you can find; raw and certified organic are the best.

If you have difficulty digesting milk (lactose intolerance is especially common among blacks, Native Americans, Mexicans, Asians, and Jews of Eastern European descent), then fermented dairy products like yogurt, kefir, buttermilk, and acidophilus milk may be more easily tolerated. You can also purchase enzymes under the trade name Lactaid to use in regular milk.

Milk: full-fat cow's milk, goat's milk, buttermilk, acidophilus milk	1 cup
Yogurt: full-fat cow's milk, plain; goat's milk, plain; kefir	1 cup

The Basic Fast Burner Eating Plan:
A Week of Sample Menus

Below are the modifications you can work with based on blood type:

- If you have Blood Type O and are lactose intolerant, try lactose-reduced dairy products that contain the enzyme product Lact-aid, or use soy cheese instead of dairy cheese, if tolerated. If you are gluten sensitive, use gluten-free breads made from rice, millet, and tapioca to replace whole wheat breads, crackers, and pita bread. Spelt and Kamut, although they contain gluten, may be better tolerated than wheat.
- Blood type A's are generally able to handle a vegetarian diet; however, if you are a type A and a fast burner, your metabolism takes precedence. You definitely need animal protein in your diet; there's just no way around it.
- Blood type B's should substitute turkey or fish for chicken in the menus, and can eat yogurt and fermented dairy products.
- Blood type AB's with more of an A food orientation should follow the A guidelines; if you lean toward B characteristics, you can add the fermented dairy products to your diet.

MONDAY

BREAKFAST:

2 Scrambled eggs with mushrooms

1 slice sprouted whole grain toast with

1 tablespoon butter

1 cup herbal tea

LUNCH:

2 ounces cold salmon salad with

1 tablespoon canola oil mayonnaise

½ cup green peas

Marinated artichoke hearts

DINNER:

4 ounces chicken liver sautéed in sherry with onions

1 Baked potato drizzled with

1 tablespoon olive oil

Steamed broccoli and cauliflower

TUESDAY

BREAKFAST:

2 ounces natural turkey sausage

½ cup home fries made with

1 tablespoon high-oleic safflower oil

1 cup herbal tea

LUNCH:

1 cup lentil soup

Steamed bok choy

1 slice sprouted whole grain toast with

1 tablespoon butter

DINNER:

4 ounces baked lobster tail with

2 teaspoons drawn butter

Green beans

1 ear corn on the cob with

1 teaspoon butter

WEDNESDAY

BREAKFAST:

Huevos rancheros made with

2 eggs, ⅓ cup pinto beans, and light tomato sauce

2 tablespoons sour cream

1 whole grain or spelt tortilla with

2 teaspoons butter

1 cup herbal tea

LUNCH:

2 ounces shrimp scampi

Warm asparagus

½ cup millet with celery and

3 tablespoon roasted pumpkin seeds

DINNER:

4 ounces roast beef

Summer squash, mushroom, and carrot medley

Spinach salad with

Bacon bits and 1 tablespoon olive oil dressing

THURSDAY

BREAKFAST:

2 ounces grilled breakfast steak

Fresh sliced tomatoes

1 slice sprouted whole rye toast with

1 tablespoon butter

1 cup herbal tea

LUNCH:

2 ounces sardines

Grated daikon radish, carrot, and chive salad with

1 tablespoon peanut oil dressing

DINNER:

4 ounces rack of lamb

1 steamed artichoke with

1 tablespoon drawn butter

½ cup brown rice

FRIDAY

BREAKFAST:

1 cup V-8 juice

2 slices Canadian bacon and

1 poached egg

1 slice sprouted whole grain toast and

1 teaspoon butter

1 cup herbal tea

LUNCH:

Cobb salad made with

2 ounces sliced dark-meat chicken, 2 ounces cheddar cheese, ½
small avocado, 5 large olives, lettuce, tomatoes, and
cucumbers

2 tablespoons ranch-style dressing made from sour cream

4 Ry-Krisp crackers

DINNER:

3 ounces spareribs

Baked cauliflower with toasted sesame seeds

½ cup green peas with

1 tablespoon butter

SATURDAY

BREAKFAST:

½ cup unsweetened cranberry juice cocktail

2 ounces Swiss cheese melted on

1 slice sprouted whole grain toast with

1 teaspoon butter

1 cup herbal tea

LUNCH:

2 chicken frankfurters on

1 whole grain bun

Cabbage slaw with

1 tablespoon olive oil and cider vinegar dressing

DINNER:

4 ounces veal cutlet

Spinach and mushrooms sautéed with

2 tablespoons high-oleic safflower oil

½ cup roasted new potatoes with parsley

SUNDAY

BREAKFAST:

2 ounces pickled herring

Stewed tomatoes

1 slice sprouted whole grain toast with

1 tablespoon butter

1 cup herbal tea

LUNCH:

2 ounces chopped liver

1 slice sprouted rye bread

Carrot and celery sticks with

1 tablespoon sesame seed butter dip (tahini)

DINNER:

4 ounces lamb medallions

Okra, stir-fried in

1 tablespoon high-oleic safflower oil

1 cup baked winter squash

- Beverages with meals include water, herbal tea (oatstraw and horsetail are best for the fast burner), Kukicha (Japanese twig tea), or coffee substitutes. One cup of coffee is okay.
- Drink at least eight glasses of pure water daily between meals. Herbal teas and coffee substitutes can be used as beverages but are not substitutes for water.
- Snacks: choose from nut butters (peanut, almond) on rice cakes or Essene bread (flourless bread), and fruit with cheese or yogurt.

Fast Burner Daily Vitamin and Mineral Supplements

In keeping with the theme of this book, a list of vitamin supplements is only recommended as a guide. Some individuals may need ten times more vitamin C, for example, than others. The vitamins in the following list act as co-factors in the energy cycles of the body, and may be of most help to the fast burner. Remember, we are all different, and we each have a unique bio-chemical blueprint. Consequently, we each have different metabolic needs. The following list should be used as a basic guide. For further guidance in personalizing your unique daily vitamin and mineral intake, please consult a qualified health practitioner.

Note: These supplements should be taken with food, once a day, unless otherwise noted.

Vitamin A—10,000 IU

Niacinamide—100 mg

Calcium pantothenate (pantothenic acid)—100 mg 3 times daily

Vitamin B$_{12}$—200 mcg

Choline—100 mg 3 times daily

Inositol—100 mg 3 times daily

Vitamin C—1,000 mg 3 times daily

Bioflavonoids—500 mg

Vitamin E—200 IU 2 times daily

Calcium—1,500 mg

Chelated zinc—20 mg

Iodine—150 mcg

MAXEPA—1,000 mg 2 times daily

How to Start

After looking over all these lists of foods, you may be feeling a bit overwhelmed, thinking you will have to make some drastic changes in your diet. The best way to start any new eating plan is to begin gradually. Start by gently increasing your daily exercise. If you lead a basically sedentary life, start walking around the block once a day, gradually increasing the amount of time and adding new activities. If you already work out three or four times a week, check this book's section on exercise to make sure you are doing activities that are best suited to your blood type.

Next, look over the food lists carefully. You might find it helpful to keep a diary of the foods you usually eat over the span of a few days or a week, noting everything you eat (including snacks, condiments, etc.) so that you can compare your usual diet with the sample plan best suited for your type. It's not easy to eliminate everything you've been eating and to add a whole list of new foods into your daily routine overnight, so start slowly. You can begin by either increasing your recommended foods, cutting back on the foods that are not recommended for your type, or a little of both.

For any type, if you eat several pieces of fruit or drink a lot of fruit juice every day, start by reducing your intake until you are down to one or two pieces a day. The same should hold true if you eat a lot of bread, pasta, bagels, muffins, and crackers: start cutting back on servings and portions, balancing them out with protein and vegetables. If you are a *slow burner,* start substituting chicken every time you would normally have a steak or a burger (especially when you eat out). Conversely, if you are a *fast burner,* try having a steak instead of pasta. A slow but deliberate pattern of increasing the recommended foods and decreasing the foods that are not recommended for your type will help you make the transition with ease.

Food for Thought

No matter what type of biochemistry you have, are you conscious of avoiding the many unnatural foods that are frequently found in so many products today? You should because the processing of these foods seems to be one of the main reasons our society has so many weight problems and so much degenerative disease.

Are you resisting the natural inclination to want to follow either the slow or fast burner's sample menu to the letter? Particularly if you know a specific food doesn't agree with you, are you honoring the signals your body gives you and freely making substitutions in the plan when necessary?

Let's say you're a fast burner with Native American ancestors from the plains area of America. Have you considered that buffalo might be a better meat for you to include in your diet in place of some of the other meats mentioned in the sample menu?

This is just one example of innovative questions you may need to ask yourself to help you personalize your diet. If you don't know about your heritage, seek out the answers from your parents and relatives. Ask them what types of foods your ancestors might have eaten. You'll learn a lot about yourself, your unique biochemistry, and the right diet for you in the process.

Remember: When we design an eating plan that's right for each of us, no two diets will ever be the same. Each diet will be as unique as each one of us, and what we need to eat for our best health is something we should never be ashamed of.

Have you given up feeling guilty or defensive about giving your body the foods it craves and needs to function at its best? You should because when you strengthen your physical self with the foods that are genetically right for you, you also will fortify your emotional, mental, and spiritual selves as well.

Closing Words

●

Hopefully, this book will not be an ending but a beginning for you. It is my desire that you use the information that has been compiled in this book as a springboard for further investigation into personalizing health. As I have said, I do not have all the answers but what I do know is that one diet does not work for everyone and each individual has to learn what works best for him or her.

Personalizing nutrition is not a simple task, as you can see. We all share some very basic common needs yet we have unique requirements as well. As I have explained, some individuals function better on an eating plan that emphasizes more protein and healthy fats while others seem to do quite well on high amounts of carbohydrates. Some people are born to be vegetarians; others are not. Men lose weight faster than women even though their exercise and calorie levels may be the same.

Many of our unique differences can be better understood when we examine the roles that our ancestry, heredity, blood type, and metabolism play in total health. These areas provide helpful clues in determining the right diet for each person. Ultimately, the past may be our greatest asset in shaping our present and future nutrition programs.

Resources: Where To Go For Help

●

Aatron Medical Services
12832 S. Chadron Avenue
Hawthorn, CA 90250
1-800-377-7744
1-800-433-9750 (in California)

A laboratory that specializes in amino acid testing by analyzing plasma and urine samples, Aatron Medical Services has trained technologists who can test for levels of 41 amino acids and analogs and will provide courtesy consultations over the phone.

American Academy of Nutrition
3408 Sausalito
Corona del Mar, CA 92625
1-800-290-4226

The American Academy of Nutrition offers nutrition education courses through home study and is the only nutrition home study school in the world that is accredited by the U.S. Department of Education's National Home Study Council. The Academy is also approved as a continuing education provider for many groups, including nurses and the American College of Sports Medicine, and is approved by the U.S. Department of Defense for military tuition assistance. As director of continuing education for the American Academy of Nutrition, I highly recommend the academy's courses for anyone who wishes to increase his or her knowledge about the fascinating subject of nutrition.

American Biologics-Mexico S.A.
1180 Walnut Avenue
Chula Vista, CA 91911
1-800-227-4458

American Biologics-Mexico S.A. Medical Center is an innovative leader in individualized, integrated metabolic programs. American Biologics has produced dramatic results in the treatment of chronic fatigue, allergies, multiple sclerosis, and a wide range of immunological diseases. It has assembled promising therapies and diagnostics from all over the world to manage degenerative diseases. It maintains North America's only center for the fresh, live cell therapy method pioneered 50 years ago by the Swiss physician Paul Niehans for regeneration and rejuvenation.

Analytical Research Labs, Inc.
8650 North 22nd Avenue
Phoenix, AZ 85021
1-602-995-1580

Analytical Research Labs, Inc., is a tissue mineral analysis laboratory developed by Dr. Paul Eck, who has spent 35 years studying how minerals affect our biochemistry and dietary needs. The results of a tissue mineral analysis from this lab can help an individual determine whether he or she is a slow burner or a fast burner.

HealthExcel, Inc.
Route 1, Box 495
Winthrop, WA 98862
1-509-996-2131

HealthExcel features a computerized comprehensive analysis of individualized metabolic typing. An evaluation consists of the following elements: hair tissue mineral analysis, body type photographs, and a special questionnaire that includes a three-day diet record; special tests; and physical, dietary, and psychological characteristics; as well as a genetic/developmental-type survey and *Candida* overgrowth self-test. This computerized system was first developed by Dr. William Donald Kelley in the 1970s and has reached its present form through the work of Bill Wolcott.

Huggins Diagnostic Center
5080 List Drive
Colorado Springs, CO 80919
1-800-331-2303

Hal Huggins, D.D.S., who is considered by many to be the top mercury toxicity expert in the country, founded this center, which specializes in diagnosing and treating heavy metal toxicity and involvement as a cause of many common health problems. For individuals who have tried countless other avenues for restoring and personalizing their health, looking at the possibility of heavy metal toxicity from dental fillings may be one more area worth investigating.

Joanie Greggains Productions
P.O. Box 2708
Sausalito, California 94966

Joanie Greggains is a highly respected fitness expert whose knowledge and understanding of the human body make her tops in the fitness field. Her videos "Joannie Greggains' Holiday Workout" and "Joanie Greggains' Classical Workout" are unique and so much fun to do. "The Holiday Workout" is accompanied by Christmas music and "The Classical Workout" is, you guessed it, accompanied by the classics. You will find both videos uplifting to body, mind, and soul.

Malter Institute for Natural Development, Inc.
Hilltop Professional Plaza
650 E. Higgins Road, Suite 5 East
Schaumburg, IL 60173
1-708-579-0220

At this institute, clinical psychologist Rick Malter, Ph.D., has put together some rather unique concepts regarding tissue mineral analysis and the oxidation types. He applies tissue mineral analysis to different types of psychological, emotional, and behavioral problems. Dr. Malter holds classes and seminars on a regular basis for professionals and the general public.

Price-Pottenger Nutrition Foundation (PPNF)
P.O. Box 2614
La Mesa, CA 91943
1-619-574-7763

This is a source that can help you locate a nutritionally oriented health care professional who can help you apply the nutrition information found in this book. Simply send a $6 donation to the address shown above. Please be sure to indicate the state for which you are requesting a referral listing.

Contact PPNF for:
• Referrals to nutritionally oriented health care professionals
• Catalog of books, audio and video tapes, slides, etc.
• Ecology, nutrition, and organic gardening resources
• Membership information
• Quarterly *PPNF Journal* and *Eco-Nutrition News*

The Price-Pottenger Nutrition Foundation is a nonprofit, tax-exempt educational organization dedicated to the promotion of enhanced health through an awareness of ecology, life-style, and healthy food production for sound nutrition. At its core are the landmark works of Drs. Weston A. Price and Francis M. Pottenger, Jr., pioneers in modern nutrition research.

Uni Key Health Systems
P.O. Box 7168
Bozeman, MT 59771
1-800-888-4353

This company is a source for the innovative and advanced natural products for chronic fatigue, candidiasis, parasite infection, and general nutritional needs. Uni Key also distributes my books *Beyond Pritikin, Super Nutrition for Women, Guess What Came to Dinner,* and *Super Nutrition for Menopause.* Ask for a brochure about all the latest products.

References

●

Abraham, Guy. "The Calcium Controversy." *Journal of Applied Nutrition* 34 (1982): 69.

Abraham, G. E., et al. "A Total Dietary Program Emphasizing Magnesium Instead of Calcium." *Journal of Reproductive Medicine* 35(5) (1990): 503–07.

Abrams, Leon H., Jr. "Anthropological Research Reveals Human Dietary Requirements for Optimal Health." *Journal of Applied Nutrition* 34(1) (1982).

Abravanel, Elliot. *Dr. Abravanel's Body Type Diet.* New York: Bantam, 1983.

Atkins, Robert. *Dr. Atkins' New Diet Revolution.* New York: Evans, 1992.

———. *Dr. Atkins' Super Energy Diet.* New York: Crown, 1976.

Balance Nutritional Manual. Santa Barbara, Calif.: Bio Foods, Inc., 1993.

Bates, Charles. *Essential Fatty Acids and Immunity in Mental Health.* Tacoma, Wash.: Life Science Press, 1987.

Bernstein, Richard, M.D. *Diabetes, Type II.* New York: Prentice Hall, 1990.

Bieler, Henry, M.D. *Food Is Your Best Medicine.* New York: Random House, 1966.

Cohen, Mark Nathan. *Health and the Rise of Civilization.* New Haven and London: Yale University Press, 1989.

Crook, William G., M. D. *The Yeast Connection, 3rd ed.* Jackson, Tenn.: Professional Books, 1986.

D'Adamo, James. *The D'Adamo Diet.* New York: McGraw-Hill, 1989.

D'Adamo, P. J., and E. R. Zampieron. "ABO Bias May Signal Innate Differences in 'Natural' Immunity." *Journal of Naturopathic Medicine* 2(1) (1991): 11–16.

191

———. "Gut Ecosystems I: Defense Mechanisms and Interactive Effects: Endotoxins, Allergens and Candidiasis." *Townsend Letters for Doctors,* April 1991.

———. "Gut Ecosystems II: Special Characteristics: Lectins and Mitogens." *Townsend Letters for Doctors,* November 1993.

———. "Gut Ecosystems III: The ABO Blood Groups and Other Polymorphic Systems." *Townsend Letters for Doctors,* August/September 1990.

Dallas, Clouatre, Ph.D. *Getting Lean With Anti-Fat Nutrients.* San Francisco: Pax Publishing, 1993.

DeSilver, Drew. "Putting Meat Back on the Menu." *Vegetarian Times,* January 1995, pp. 67–72.

Diamond, H., and M. Diamond. *Fit for Life.* New York: Warner Books, 1985.

"Do Our Genes Determine Which Foods We Should Eat?" *Newsweek,* August 9, 1993, p. 64.

Eating Right Pyramid. USDA Food Plan, Human Nutrition Service, Leaflet 572, August 1992.

Eaton, S. Boyd, M.D., Marjorie Shostak, and Melvin Konner, M.D. *The Paleolithic Prescription.* New York: Harper & Row, 1988.

Enig, Mary, Ph.D. *Trans-Fatty Acids in the Food Supply: A Comprehensive Report Covering 60 Years of Research.* Silver Spring, Md.: Enig Associates, 1993.

Erasmus, Udo. *Fats and Oils.* Burnaby, B.C., Canada: Alive Books, 1992.

Ezrin, Calvin, and R. Kowalski. *The Endocrine Control Diet.* (New York: Harper & Row, 1990.

"Fat Times." *Time,* January 16, 1995, pp. 58–95.

Finnegan, John. *The Facts about Fats.* Berkeley, Calif.: Celestial Arts, 1993.

Galbo, H. "Endocrinology and Metabolism in Exercise." *International Journal of Sports Medicine* 2 (1981): 125–30.

Gittleman, Ann Louise, M. S. *Super Nutrition for Menopause.* New York: Pocket Books, 1993.

———. *Guess What Came to Dinner.* Garden City, N.Y.: Avery, 1993.

———. *Super Nutrition for Women.* New York: Bantam Books, 1991.

Grunwald, Lisa. "28 Questions about Fat." *Life,* February 1995, pp. 58–74.

Guyton, Arthur C. *Textbook of Medical Physiology, 8th ed.* Philadelphia: W.B. Saunders Co., 1991.

HealthExcel. "H.O.P.E. Report." HealthExcel Inc., 1986.

Heller, Richard, and Rachel Heller. *Carbohydrate Addicts Diet.* New York: NAL Dutton, 1992.

Hills, Hilda. *Good Food, Gluten Free.* New Canaan, Conn.: Keats, 1976.

Hunter, Beatrice. *Gluten Intolerance.* New Canaan, Conn.: Keats, 1987.

"Insulin Resistance—A Secret Killer?" *New England Journal of Medicine* 320(1), March 16, 1989, pp. 733–34.

Jenkins, D. J. A., et al. "Glycemic Index of Foods: A Physiological Basis for Carbohydrate Exchange." *American Journal of Clinical Nutrition* 34 (1981): 362–366.

Kelley, W. D. *The Metabolic Types.:* Kelley Foundation, 1976.

Kushi, Michio. *Healing Through Macrobiotics.* Tokyo and New York: Japan Publications, 1978.

Lad, Vasant. *Ayurveda: The Science of Self Healing.* Santa Fe, N. Mex.: Lotux Press, 1984.

Malter, R. F. "Energy, Stress and the New Nutrition: New Concepts for Understanding Today's Health Trends," *unpublished paper.* Schuaumburg, Ill.: *Malter Institute for Natural Development, Inc.,* 1993.

Moore Lappé, Frances. *Diet for a Small Planet.* New York: Ballentine, 1971.

Mourant, A. E. *Blood Groups and Diseases.* Oxford: Oxford University Press, 1978.

Newbold, H. L., M.D. *Dr. Newbold's A Type-B Type Weight Loss Book.* (New Canaan, Conn.: Keats, 1991.

Ornish, Dean. *Eat More Weigh Less.* New York: HarperCollins, 1993.

Page, Melvin E., and H. Leon Abrams, Jr. *Your Body Is Your Best Doctor.* New Canaan, Conn.: Keats, 1972.

———. *Body Chemistry in Health and Disease.* Biochemical Research Foundation, 1949. (Reprinted by Price-Pottenger Nutrition Foundation, La Mesa, Calif.)

———. *Degeneration-Regeneration.* Biochemical Research Foundation, 1949. (Reprinted by Price-Pottenger Nutrition Foundation, La Mesa, Calif.)

Passwater, Richard A., Ph.D. "An Interview with Mary Enig. Ph.D.: Health Risks from Processed Foods and Trans Fats." *Whole Foods,* January 1994, pp. 47–52.

———. "An Interview with Mary Enig. Ph.D.: Health Risks from Processed Foods and Trans Fats, Part II." *Whole Foods,* December 1993, pp. 52–56.

———. "An Interview with Mary Enig. Ph.D.: Health Risks from Processed Foods and Trans Fats, Part III." *Whole Foods,* November 1993, pp. 46–51.

"Position for the American Dietetic Association: Vegetarian Diets." *Journal of the American Dietetic Association,* November 1993, pp. 1317–1318.

Pottenger, Francis M., Jr., M.D. *Pottenger's Cats.* La Mesa, Calif.: Price-Pottenger Nutrition Foundation, 1983.

Powter, Susan. *Stop the Insanity.* New York: Simon & Schuster, 1993.

Pritikin, Nathan. *Live Longer Now.* New York: Grosset & Dunlap, 1974.

Pritikin, Nathan. *Pritikin Program for Diet and Exercise.* New York: Grosset & Dunlap, 1979.

————. "High Carbohydrate Diets: Maligned and Misunderstood." *Journal of Applied Nutrition,* Winter, 1976.

Quillen, Patrick. *La Costa Book of Nutrition.* New York: Pharos, 1988.

Reading, Chris, M.D., and Ross S. Meillon. *Your Family Tree Connection.* New Canaan, Conn.: Keats, 1988.

Reaven, G. M. "Role of Insulin Resistance in Human Disease." *Diabetes* 37 (1988): 1595–1607.

Roberts, H. J., M.D. *Sweet'ner Dearest.* West Palm Beach, Fla.: Sunshine Sentinel Press, 1992.

Rosenvold, Lloyd. *Can a Gluten-Free Diet Help.* New Canaan, Conn.: Ketas, 1992.

Scheer, James S. "Supplements Fill Gaps in Vegetarian Diets." *Nutrition for Today's Living,* August 1994, pp. 43–45.

Schmid, Ronald F., N.D. *Native Nutrition: Eating According to Ancestral Wisdom.* Rochester, Vt.: Healing Arts Press 1987, revised 1994.

Sears, Barry, Ph.D. "Essential Fatty Acids and Dietary Endocrinology: A Hypothesis for Cardiovascular Treatment." *Journal of Advancement in Medicine* 6 (Winter 1993): 211–224.

————. "Why You're Still Fat." *Let's Play Magazine,* November 1991, p. 12.

Sheats, Cliff. *Lean Bodies.* Fort Worth, Tex.: Summit Group, 1992.

Shelton, Herbert M., Ph.D. *Fasting Can Save Your Life.* Chicago: Natural Hygiene Press, 1971.

————. *Principles of Natural Hygiene.* San Antonio, Tex.: Dr. Shelton's Health School, 1964.

————. *Natural Hygiene, Man's Pristine Way of Life.* San Antonio, Tex.: Dr. Shelton's Health School, 1968.

Smith, Lendon H., M.D., *Happiness Is a Healthy Life.* (New Canaan, Conn.: Keats Publishing, Inc., 1992.

Toshitaka, Nomi, and Alexander Besher. *You Are Your Blood Type.* New York: Pocket Books, 1983.

Vagnini, Frederic J. "Syndrome X—Triglycerides, Insulin Resistance, Hypertension and Cardiovascular Disease." *NY Hospital & Health News* 7 (1992). 2–3.

Valletta, D. J., et al. "Effects of Low and High Carbohydrate Supplemented Diets and Running Performance." *Department of Sports Medicine, Pepperdine University, Sports Medicine, Training and Rehabilitation* 4 (4), December 1993.

Watson, George. *Nutrition and Your Mind.* New York: Harper & Row, 1972.

Webb, Denise. "Nutritionists Make Predictions about Food, Health Issues for '94." *The New Mexican,* December 29, 1993.

Weston, Price. *Nutrition and Physical Degeneration.* Price-Pottenger Foundation, 1945. New Canaan, Conn.: Keats, 1989.

Wiley, Rudolf. *BioBalance.* Tacoma, Wash.: Life Sciences Press, 1989.

Williams, Roger, Ph.D. *Nutrition Against Disease.* New York: Bantam, 1973.

———. *Nutrition in a Nutshell.* New York: Doubleday, 1962.

———. *Biochemical Individuality.* New York: Wiley and Sons, 1956.

Wolever, T. M. S. "Relationship Between Dietary Fiber Content and Composition in Foods and the Glycemic Index." *American Journal of Clinical Nutrition* 51 (1990): 72–75.

Yudkin, John, M.D. *Sweet and Dangerous.* New York: Bantam Books, 1972.

Zabaroin, Ivana, et al. "Risk Factors for Coronary Artery Disease in Healthy Persons with Hyperinsulinism and Normal Glucose Tolerance." *New England Journal of Medicine* 302 (1989): 702–706.

Zucker, Martin. "What's Gumming Up Your Works?" *Let's Live,* February 1983, pp. 79–81.

Index

About the Authors

—

ANN LOUISE GITTLEMAN, M.S. and Certified Nutrition Specialist, is one of America's leading nutritionists. She is the author of many best-selling books, including *Super Nutrition for Menopause* and *Beyond Pritikin*. She is the recipient of the prestigious Excellence in Medical Communications Award and is a Nutrition Director of the American Academy of Nutrition.

•

JAMES WILLIAM TEMPLETON is a teacher, researcher, and formulator of nutritional products for the natural foods industry. His personal health story is featured in several books, including *Cancer-Free* (Japan Publications).

•

CANDELORA VERSACE is an award-winning journalist based in Santa Fe, New Mexico, whose coverage of arts and culture appears regularly in several publications. Her book, *Refining the Vision: The Art World of Santa Fe,* is scheduled for release in late 1995 by Penny Whistle Press.